The Vegan FIGHT

Good Health is a Gift

WHITNEY PEOPLES

Library of Congress Number: 2020901627

ISBN: 978-1-7345655-0-8 (Ebook)

ISBN: 978-1-7345655-1-5 (Paperback)

Acknowledgements

The information in this book was written with love and genuine concern for future generations. It is partly based on my views and personal experiences as a vegan. There are findings on vegan historical events and dieting that have been cited and referenced. I apologize in advance if I inadvertently failed to credit the originator on the material used.

The Vegan Fight:

Are steps to conquer yourself rather than losing yourself trying to conquer a world that supports an unhealthy way of living.

*My own view is that being a vegetarian or vegan is not an end in itself,
but a means towards reducing both human and animal suffering and
leaving a habitable planet to future generations.*
~ Peter Singer

*Even when we can't see exactly how our actions make a difference,
sometimes it's enough to do something just because it's the right thing to do.*
~ Colleen Patrick-Goudreau

*The vegan movement is one of the fastest growing social justice
movements in the world today.*
~ Melanie Joy

Contents

Part One

What It Means To Live A Vegan Lifestyle

Part Two

What It Means To Live A Healthy Lifestyle

Part Three

How To Find The Balance

Breaking Barriers for The Almighty Vegan Fight

"If nature didn't make it, don't take it."

~ Dr. Sebi

Veganism!? Who would consider a lifestyle free of meat and dairy? Growing up in South Carolina, all I wanted was Little Debbie cakes (oatmeal pies, strawberry swiss rolls, and nutty bars). I had no idea what it meant to be vegan. I didn't see it as a diet or a new health wave. I thought it was a lifestyle that required esoteric wisdom that only important people had the power to master. Someone from my upbringing wouldn't know where to begin to grasp veganism, nor would they want to go against everything passed down from generation to generation. Who would be crazy enough to turn down mom's secret recipe to her famous casserole or grandma's homemade biscuits?

I have come to realize that taste alone perpetuated this unhealthy way of living. As ignorant as I was about dieting, I don't think I heard the term vegan or veganism until I enrolled in college. I started to meet people from different backgrounds where being health conscious was normal. Being educated about veganism was an eye opening experience because I really didn't have a clue. I would read up on it almost every day but couldn't find a straight answer on how to sustain it. The idea of only eating fruits, beans, and vegetables (with no fast food options!) scared the crap out of me. I convinced myself that veganism was for people who wanted to lose weight and I was satisfied with my body and the curves that came with it. Once I overcame my own ignorance, I began to study the truth about the human body and what we should be eating to support our bodily functions. My thoughts on everything I've learned revealed the lack of accountability by society for the adverse effects of consuming animal products.

Without question, a vegan diet that relies on whole foods rather than meat and dairy alternatives provides the most health benefits. Among the many vegan diets, two things remain consistent, they are eco-friendly and cruelty-free. The health benefits between them differ. An ultra-processed vegan diet does not share the same nutritional value as a whole-foods, vegan diet. While they are tasty, satisfying, and convenient, they expose you to the same terminal diseases as any meat eating diet. Ultra-processed foods contain several ingredients that make them appealing and attractive to buyers, including high-fructose corn syrup. Building a healthy relationship with food will help break common addictions formed by ingredients such as salt and sugar.

Putting a label on your dietary choices doesn't automatically guarantee a healthy relationship with food. A self-educated vegan has a better chance at maintaining this lifestyle than someone jumping in with unrealistic expectations. A frivolous reason such as a desire to lose weight is a setup to lose your fight before you begin. It's important to understand why you are transitioning and if veganism is capable of meeting your expectations. The most effective way to start a vegan diet is by adding more vegan options to your daily meals. Once you're comfortable, slowly replace meat with plant protein until you're comfortable enough to remove meat and dairy completely from your diet. Keep in mind that the fight is within you. Veganism is not always an accepted lifestyle especially for families that use food as a huge part of holiday celebrations and religious gatherings. Be prepared to accept the criticism for your decision to transition even when it's coming from people you love. If you have a bigger goal in mind and if you are using veganism to master the physical aspect of healthy living, then holistic practices maybe something you want to consider.

Holistic living covers many areas of your life and requires some level of knowledge. Veganism is not a type of change that focuses on your mental, emotional, and spiritual health. It is a type of lifestyle that is capable of improving your physical health. Take time to explore veganism and see what it has to offer, and then choose a vegan diet that best suits you.

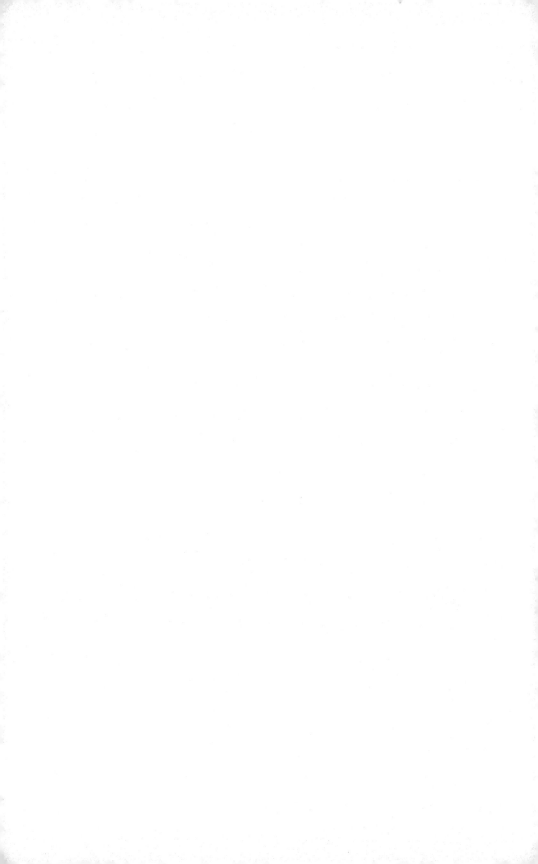

Part One

What It Means To Live A Vegan Lifestyle

Chapter 1

Transitioning to Veganism

"In my food world, there is no fear or guilt, only joy and balance."
~ Ellie Krieger

Transitioning to a vegan diet is not as complicated as it seems. Having little to no knowledge about the diet may cause doubts to linger, and that could be daunting. View it as a process and don't be too hard on yourself. You will fail and you will unknowingly eat foods that are made with animal products. It takes patience and dedication to master something that is completely opposite of what you're accustomed to.

The first step you may want to take in any process is to question your decision. Yes, question it! If you're not passionate and serious about your decision, no one else will be. It's important to note that what happens in the heart and mind eventually manifest on the outside, so it's impossible to hide those inner feelings. If you want to get all the support you need from family and friends, you should have a level of seriousness about it. You don't want to be taken as a joke and live a life being pressured to eat non-vegan foods because no one respects your decision. After making peace with your new journey, make it clear to the people in your daily life. For some people, this could be the most difficult step in the entire process.

Feeling inspired to explore veganism is one aspect of the transitioning process, but the doubts created from common misconceptions have led some beginners astray. What's worse than debating a topic with someone whose information comes from nothing more than a brief conversation with a non-vegan restaurant chef who has no desire to cater to vegans? Or, from someone who abandoned their vegan diet because it required too much work and decided to discourage others from considering the lifestyle? I compiled seven popular misconceptions about veganism, and debunked them with hopes of changing your views about the lifestyle.

Misconception 1: A Vegan Diet Is Expensive

Opting for an ultra-processed vegan diet can be expensive. If your desire is to replace meat, eggs, and milk with vegan alternatives, then yes, you can expect it to be costly. If you haven't taken the time to read up on maintaining a vegan diet, you may start by comparing prices. You will discover that vegan eggs, vegan sausage links, and dairy-free mayonnaise are much more expensive than chicken eggs, pork sausage, and dairy mayonnaise. This misconception will then be proven to you as a fact. You will immediately become discouraged and decide that you can't afford to change your diet. I am here to tell you that veganism doesn't have to be expensive.

A plant-only diet that consists of primarily fruits, vegetables, legumes, and whole grains is much less expensive than a diet consisting of meat and dairy. Prior to transitioning to veganism, I spent more money on a pescatarian diet than I ever spent on a plant-only diet. Every vegan has a preference: some people desire a gluten-free and/or non-GMO diet, while others prefer organic, whole foods, raw vegan diet. Today, there are a variety of vegan options available. Similar to meat-based diets, the cost of maintaining a vegan diet varies in price – according to the consumer's preference.

Misconception 2: A Vegan Diet Causes Protein Deficiency

This is one of the top three misconceptions especially in the fitness community. I was surprised to see the amount of fitness trainers who advised I wouldn't be able to gain as much muscle on a vegan diet. This is false! Plant-only protein is more sustainable and healthier than ingesting animal based protein. The truth is as the world population continues to increase; there won't be enough resources to sustain a meat eating diet. Over the next two decades, fish alone will be near extinction due to climate change and high demand.[1]

The most reliable source of protein is plant protein. All plants on earth contain protein. In fact, more than 13% of all plant calories are protein. Even on the strictest diet, a vegan would still be able to get the amount of protein recommended daily. The true misconception about protein is how much we believe we need per day. It is almost impossible to be protein deficient without being calorie deficient as well.[2]

Misconception 3: Honey is Vegan

Vegans like to avoid this highly divisive topic of how honey should be classified. Some vegan bloggers with a large audience have publicly spoken on this topic advising that avoiding honey is optional

---

[1] A study by Boris Worm, PhD (marine ecologist and research professor), from Dalhousie University in Halifax, Nova Scotia
[2] Saknas Halmstad, Sweden, *Protein deficiency – a rare nutrient deficiency*, (PubMed.gov: 2019)

and is usually a problem for those who wish to be true advocates for bringing an end to animal cruelty and environmental degradation.[3]

The issue on this topic has a great deal to do with the constant changes within The Vegan Society on what is acceptable in the vegan diet. An article in Vegan Society Today (2016) titled *Honey Is Not Considered Vegan, but It Is a Minor Issue for Most Vegans* - addressed how honey has been a topic of debate since the inception of veganism. The dietary definitions for whether honey is vegan have changed 10 times. These definitions have allowed honey to be consumed for a total of 30 years; however, these 30 years were never consecutive. For 14 years (1957-1962), honey was left to the discretion of the dieter. After 14 years, The Vegan Society decided to ban honey, and then made another 14-year exception in 1974. The expectation became cloudy but due the strong values and beliefs of animal activists, honey was officially declared to be a non-vegan product in 1988.[4]

Veganism was not always a driving force for the animal rights movement. There were people who wanted it to be, but health was the driving force that attracted members to The Vegan Society. Because of internal fights among members and leadership, there were changes that went against prior regulations. Depending upon who was in office, the definitions changed, which left a lot of people in a state of confusion. Being an advocate for honey in the vegan community has caused more intense debates with animal activists than most could imagine. Promoting the health benefits of a vegan diet is acceptable, but when honey becomes a topic of discussion, animal activists are ready to oppose.

People who choose veganism for health reasons claim that honey is a healthy sweetener full of vitamins and minerals. However, the body

---

[3] *Is Honey Vegan? A Look at the Debate*, Mama Sezz: 2019, url
https://www.mamasezz.com/blogs/news/is-honey-vegan
[4] *Honey is not Considered Vegan; it is a Minor Issue for Most Vegans*. Vegan Society Today: 2016, url: http://vegansociety.today/honey.html

processes honey the same as white sugar, so nothing significantly different is happening in how the body processes them both. Whether you're choosing veganism to improve your health or to support animal rights, consumption of honey doesn't benefit either agenda.

Misconception 4: You'll Lose Weight on a Vegan Diet

Non-vegans presume vegans are healthy and fit, but that's often false. If you're on an ultra-processed vegan diet containing refined sugar, unhealthy fats, and simple carbs with an outrageous amount of sodium, your chances of losing weight is at an all-time low. The body responds to ultra-processed foods based on factors outside of your dietary preference. The body doesn't check to see if the processed food contains animal products to ensure there are no negative effects. The best way to understand this is to view milk and meat as an ingredient rather than as a product. For example, you cannot make a cookie out of milk alone. There are several other ingredients involved. The only difference between a vegan cookie and a non-vegan cookie is one to two ingredients; if you substitute the cow's milk with a milk alternative (almond milk, soymilk, coconut milk, etc.), the cookie will still look and taste the same. The unhealthy ingredients will remain because it's not the milk that ruins the cookie's nutritional value, it's also the sugar and other unhealthy ingredients that result in fat storage and health challenges.

Diseases and fat-inducing foods are not limited to animal products. Meat and dairy is not the culprit of most health problems. Yes, it has been proven that a healthy whole foods vegan diet consisting primarily of fruits and vegetables is conducive to maintaining homeostasis, but so does any minimally processed flexitarian diet.[5] Thousands of men and women compete in body-building competitions that thrive on

---

[5] Flexitarian Diet: Vegetarian diet with much less meat

meat-eating diets. If your goal is to reach optimal health, then you should look far beyond veganism and do your research on fat-forming foods, processed foods, and ultra-processed foods. You'll discover that a plant-only diet is the best approach to dieting.

Misconception 5: My 95-Year Old Grandmother Has Been Eating Meat All Her Life

I hear this much too often, but no one ever mentions the health complications their loved ones may face at this stage in their life. One individual compared to a whole population is not enough to prove anything. The point is not to discuss the death rates for those who eat meat, but the health complications people face when eating a large amount of meat and dairy products. Individuals who primarily thrive on a plant-only diet have a longer life expectancy without having to rely on pharmaceutical medicine than those who eat a large amount of meat and dairy products.[6] Your grandmother is blessed to see 95 years of her life, but are those years as pleasant as they could be? How many years did she enjoy in her older age where health complications didn't intervene? Living in misery and being restricted from certain activities due to health complications is barely living at all. Have you ever heard the popular saying that *Health is Wealth*? It's true! Without your good health, nothing else matters because you can't enjoy the luxuries you have due to complications that money can't fix. If you want to obtain optimal health, do it the right way. Stop trying to create a path to live a healthy happy life while eating unhealthy foods.

---

[6] *Why Do Vegans Live Longer?* Food & Living Vegan, url:
https://www.veganfoodandliving.com/why-do-vegans-live-longer/ (accessed: December 3, 2019).

Misconception 6: Vegans Have to Supplement Their Diets With Vitamins

It takes little to no effort to adopt a nutrient-dense vegan diet without having to use dietary supplements. For example, if you lack vitamin D, spend more time outside allowing your body to produce it. A vitamin D deficiency is not caused by adopting a vegan diet. Some things just happen and the climate has a lot to do with it. Here's a short story during my meat-eating days that will help you put things into perspective. After years of eating whatever I wanted, I went to the doctor for my yearly physical just to discover I was severely deficient in vitamin D. I was prescribed 50,000 iu to take once per week and given the directive to return at the end of the fourth week to have my vitamin D level tested again. Normal vitamin D levels range from 30-50 ng/ml; I was at 11 ng/ml. Attempting to raise my level was a journey within itself, but I am a living example that your diet is not the underlying cause of a deficiency.

The leading dietary concern that raises eyebrows is the risk of a vitamin B-12 deficiency. People who are suffering from B-12 deficiency are not all vegan. Stomach protein allows our body to absorb B-12 from the food we eat. When our body is not producing enough stomach protein, this could cause us to become vitamin B-12 deficient. This could happen to anyone, regardless of diet. However, I do recommend new vegans to pay closer attention to their food combination to avoid foods that do not provide the necessary vitamins and minerals needed to maintain a healthy lifestyle.

Pointing out the disadvantages of adopting a vegan diet only highlights how we've been misinformed. In fact, non-vegans are often deficient in more vitamins and minerals than vegans. Just to list a few: non-vegans are commonly deficient in magnesium, calcium, vitamin C, and folate (B vitamin). Since we live in a time aimed to decrease sanitation issues, we're advised that the cheapest and most reliable source of vitamin B-12 is animal products. However, meat fecal contamination is currently at an all-time high, which is why untreated river/lake water is not a reliable source of B-12.[7] Meat and dairy should not be advertised as a healthy and sustainable source of B-12 since it causes long-term damage to the human body. Recent studies suggest that supplementing is the best reliable source for B-12 for everyone.[8]

Misconception 7: It's Unhealthy to Be Vegan While Pregnant

My friends and I decided to start our vegan journey together. After a few months, one of my friends became pregnant and became concerned if veganism was the best choice. There were questions pertaining to her nutrient intake and whether she was getting enough vitamins and minerals to ensure a healthy newborn. Just two months into her pregnancy, she decided to discontinue her journey to veganism and add meat and dairy back to her diet until the baby was born. When I asked why, she said her doctor believed it was best for her. I immediately became furious. What type of doctor tells their patient a meat-eating diet is best instead of advising the best vegan food options to ensure a healthy pregnancy? It is critical to adhere to a whole foods plant-only diet especially in the first trimester to avoid any complications in your pregnancy; however, veganism itself does not provide additional risks to pregnancy.

A whole foods vegan diet is a healthy lifestyle, not a gamble you take at the risk of your child's mental and physical development. Using nuts, seeds, legumes, and grains for iron and replacing whole

[7] Kimberly Kindy, *Customers are buying contaminated meat, doctors' group says in lawsuit*, The Washington Post: 2019.
[8] *Why It's Not Just a Vegan Issue*, Rise of the Vegan: 2017, url: https://www.riseofthevegan.com/blog/b12-is-not-just-a-vegan-problem

milk with coconut milk are reliable substitutions. It's important to combine the right type of foods to optimize each meal. Eating veggies with some melons and berries on the side for vitamin C are minor changes that offer a whole lot of benefits. The first recommendation made by your doctor is to start taking prenatal vitamins. This is recommended for all women expecting, not just women that are on a vegan diet. How many cases have you heard of with a vegan diet causing birth defects? I'm sure your answer is none. Don't take on stress by allowing yourself to become consumed with the opinions of an inexperienced doctor. Get a second opinion or speak with a nutritionist who is well-versed on the lifestyle. Gather the facts before making a sound decision. Also, choose an OB-GYN who will cater to your needs instead of taking an easier route by recommending what's familiar to them.

Killing the Urge

Now that we've addressed a few common misconceptions, the transitioning process is the next big challenge to overcome. View your transition to veganism as a process rather than an all-at-once plunge. Your transition journey might include challenges like deterioration, discouragement, and isolation. Anticipating these challenges will help you get through tough times. Patience is needed and exploration, awareness, and health-consciousness are irreplaceable aspects to a new life. Try not to set expiration dates as if it's a daunting prerequisite to the vegan lifestyle – make it fun! Try cooking foods you've never tasted before and slowly remove meat and dairy by-products from your meals. Prior to embarking on my journey, butternut squash, eggplants, jackfruit, and Brussels sprouts were foods that were never introduced to me as a kid or as a meat-eating adult. I was amazed at how much I enjoyed them. I never thought Brussels sprouts would become a main ingredient in one of my famous household dishes.

We can be stubborn when it comes to our diet, but we don't have to make it difficult. The next time you're out eating with friends or family, try looking at the vegan options on the menu. Take it even further by making a vegan version of your favorite meal and see how you like it. I grew up on hotdogs and cheeseburgers. You can bet your last dollar I had no intentions on giving up those foods forever. Although I prefer a whole foods plant-only diet, I still consume processed vegan food in moderation. One thing I've learned on this journey is that permanently depriving yourself of foods you enjoy will cause you to develop a bad relationship with food and make you believe that the lifestyle is impossible to manage. The key to success is to explore healthier versions of the foods you love and eat them in moderation if your objective is to live a healthy lifestyle.

I'll never forget scrolling down my Instagram feed and reading a post about Slutty Vegan, a famous vegan restaurant in Atlanta, Georgia. The restaurant was acknowledged by several meat-eating celebrities such as rapper Da Brat, DISH Atlanta radio host and TV personality Porsha Williams, and R&B singer Usher as having one of the best cheeseburgers in town. I was reaching my one-year anniversary of veganism when I found myself standing in the Slutty Vegan truck line for an hour for a *One Night Stand* vegan burger. I heard so much about them that I had to see what the hype was about. When I took my first bite I knew that being vegan wasn't so bad after all. It felt as if my taste buds were experiencing a meat-eating flashback from the cookout days at my Auntie Sallie's house. I remember scuffing down a cheeseburger and watching my dad from the screen door flip the chicken over on the grill while I patiently waited for him to bring them inside – I was nostalgic at the least. I longed for that fulfillment of joy when the concoction of the different flavors from the burger secured my inner peace. At that moment, I had no doubt in my mind when I craved something such as a cheeseburger; I actually had vegan options to suppress those urges.

Although some people choose to slowly transition to veganism, if you feel bold and confident enough to go cold turkey, go for it! I went cold turkey and never looked back. However, the last thing I want to do is inflict my beliefs on you if you don't have the will power to successfully transition. Going cold turkey can be challenging unless your beliefs and values overpower your urges to indulge. The only reason I decided to go cold turkey was because I was experiencing health complications related to fibromyalgia. I could not shake the pain and nothing my doctor prescribed worked. I had exhausted all my options (so I thought) until I read stories on how people used their diet to cure themselves. Dieting was the common denominator of all the stories I read about people who successfully managed to reverse fibromyalgia. The top two diet recommendations were fasting/juicing and a fully raw (plant-only) vegan diet. Some mentioned Dr. Sebi's approach, which I'll be discussing in part 2 of this book, but even mentioning his approach, they all recommended a raw plant-only diet. I knew my only chance to feel physical relief was to go cold turkey.

I'm sure most of you are thinking, "How did you go cold turkey? I thought you transitioned." When I speak about my transition journey, I'm speaking about my journey from being a temporary raw vegan to reach optimal health, to a fully committed vegan who made a permanent lifestyle change for a bigger purpose. Although health was my primary reason for exploring veganism, I began to educate myself on how the world was suffering because of the food we eat, and I became concerned about our animals and environment.

Being a new vegan can be nerve wracking. Taking multivitamins at the start of your journey will ease a lot of the concerns regarding your nutrient intake. Although supplements are not mandatory, they can alleviate stress since most novices aren't aware of their source of vitamins and minerals. Most people take multivitamins anyway (which is fine!), but if you aren't taking them and you're new to veganism, you may want to consider the option. Exploring new foods and not knowing the nutritional benefits can potentially result in vitamin deficiencies. This isn't particularly a major concern for meat-eaters since our school system is designed to educate all students on animal sources for nutrients.

Plant-only sources for vitamins and minerals are not a primary concern or mandatory to be taught in schools so it's common to be unaware of your vegan options. It's perfectly normal not to know everything about vegan diets, so don't be too prideful in thinking you don't need assistance. You could be eating a large quantity of healthy foods and still not get what your body needs daily. Understanding this process is critical to effectively tailor your meals to meet your needs. Take into consideration that although meat eaters may have a varied diet which is a wide variety of foods from the five food groups (grains, dairy, fruit, vegetable, and protein), that doesn't imply that their food options are reliable sources, or even healthy.

Any dietary practices outside of the typical meat-eating American diet will come with disadvantages to some extent. When I was a kid, infomercials highlighted the benefits of meat, milk, eggs, and orange juice. When I was in school, nutrition courses did the same. Since birth, everything about the typical meat-eating American diet was instilled in me. I didn't stand a chance with learning or exploring anything outside of my norm until I was an adult. This type of education could make a person believe that other diets aren't effective, and promotes the idea that dietary alternatives aren't sustainable. We've been brainwashed our entire lives by people who were brainwashed their entire lives. The chances of anyone concluding otherwise based on a conversation or a few research studies are slim.

Limited Knowledge

Many governments aim to control its citizens. The American government in particular, has been utilizing propaganda for decades, implementing strategies to control what we think. Having the ability to change the value system of a group of people, or citizens is remarkably powerful. When it comes to the American diet, the USDA presents biased information on what we should include in our diet, and how to sustain it. To make life easier for ourselves, we soak up all the information like a sponge, failing to realize it's a broken system we entrust. Because of the evolution of technology, we have access to multiple search engines, which allow us to research the foods we eat to make better food choices. We know the information is out there, but we rely on the government to shove it down our throats. Even worse than that, we raise our children to follow the food pyramid recommended by the USDA. The food pyramid for our children is egregious. It perpetuates the idea that our children must include a small percentage of sweets (junk food) to sustain a balanced diet. Introducing problematic foods to a child's diet sets the trajectory of their eating habits. It's impossible for our children to crave unhealthful foods loaded with sugar if they were never introduced to it. Fruits contain natural fruit sugars that are sufficient for our children. Although the food groups recommended were concerning, it was the last thing I noticed on the pyramid. Nothing stood out more than the disturbing photo used for the meat group (figure 1). The audacity to use a little girl walking a dog is insensitive at the least. Using images and slogans to equate animals to food are ways to control our attitude and interests.[9]

---

[9] *Food Guide Pyramid for Young Children*, U.S. Department of Agriculture: 2014, url:https://www.fns.usda.gov/FGP4Children

Figure 1:

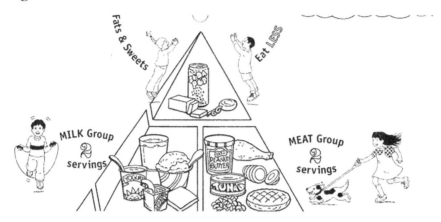

Our behavior and thoughts are learned behavior and thoughts. If we were taught how to sustain a plant-only diet, there wouldn't be a need to discuss the benefits. The investment placed upon us is so powerful that those who were born into veganism see the impact of how this world supports this one way of living on several different influential platforms. Because of technological changes along with bad leadership, people have become lazy and dependent upon those outlets for direction. No one wants to conduct their own research to challenge the status quo.

Striving to overcome the inability to think for ourselves should be a key priority in all aspects of our lives, particularly in those aspects that involve our health. It can be tough challenging everything that has been taught to us as children, but we have to think for ourselves and discover everything there is to know about the lifestyle we want to live. When we start our day by awakening our mind on what's happening in the world, we'll begin to see how everything is affected by the food we eat. This includes mental and physical challenges along with environmental degradation and animal welfare.

The law of attraction teaches us to focus on the things that positively impact our lives to set us on a path to achieve our goals. Once you decide that you're ready to transition to veganism, create your own authentic journey that complements your new lifestyle. You should surround yourself with vegans, attend vegan events that support the lifestyle, and bring awareness to loved ones who aren't familiar with veganism. If you are not able to become 100% vegan, it's perfectly fine! You don't have to express your feelings on where you are in your journey to get approval from others to move forward. Most of the things I learned weren't until my second year of being fully committed to the lifestyle. Does it get tough? Absolutely! That's why you should make the decision to transition for the right reasons. It could be ethical or religious reasons, but make sure it's something meaningful to you. If your reason isn't important, then the urge to fight through tough times won't be either. Keep a positive attitude, know why it matters to you, and plan accordingly.

The resources available to us are unlimited. There are cookbooks, transition guides, documentaries, articles, webinars, etc. The list goes on. Whatever you need is researchable and available. If you know someone who is vegan, ask questions. Don't be afraid to put yourself out there. We all had to start somewhere and although our journeys are different, no journey is perfect.

Along your journey, you may run into Cross vegans who are unreasonable and uncompromising. I refer to them as Cross vegans because Leslie J. Cross was a member of The Vegan Society who fought to redefine veganism. Cross vegans are known to take extreme, violent, and illegal action to prevent animal cruelty. Most attacks are triggered by working in the meat industry or simply being a non-vegan. However, claiming to be vegan, but failing to live by their set of values, could be a trigger for them. Fortunately, being attacked by a Cross vegan isn't a major concern for individuals who are not in the public eye. This doesn't exclude anyone from having an unpleasant experience when interacting with a Cross vegan, but it's not a lifestyle where you're continuously being scrutinized for how you live your life as a vegan. Encountering this type of attack is sometimes inevitable. I will provide more information on Cross's role in The Vegan Society in chapter 2.

Once you successfully transition, go celebrate! To master something that takes a lot of self-discipline is a big deal. You have officially set an example for someone else to be encouraged to embark on this journey. Be proud and remember where you started. Not everyone will be as strong-minded and dedicated as you are. Lead with a welcoming attitude and help others on their journey. I was once told that people who have the will power to control what they eat are capable of changing the world.

Physical, Mental, and Emotional Change

Experiencing significant bodily changes may take time depending on your diet. Don't expect a sudden boost of energy, bowel movement/ digestive changes, or weight loss overnight. To see this type of change in a short period of time depends on the type of vegan diet you choose. If you opt for processed foods, you may not see changes at all. You may experience gastrointestinal upheaval but nothing too alarming. If you want to see drastic improvement in your overall health, a whole foods vegan diet would be ideal to see that type of change. Some people who transition for health purposes also practice other healthy habits. These habits align with a holistic approach that focuses on you as a whole. I will discuss the holistic approach further in part 2 of this book.

Chapter 2

The Fight in the Vegan Community

"Winning and losing isn't everything.
Sometimes, the journey is just as important as the outcome."
~ Alex Morgan

Veganism sometimes carries a label that says – we're a group of belligerent individuals with unrelenting hostility toward people who are not interested in the lifestyle. Being a firm believer of law of attraction and its magnetic power, I know the universe grants us the same energy we expend. The absurd idea that a person would want to transition after being maligned and antagonized is an idea derived from unsettled minds. A negative reaction isn't the creation of a positive outcome. The pleasure I had with a high vibrating gem in the flesh, was more empowering than discouraging. I admired her lifestyle, but not enough to want to transition. If anything, it was curiosity that captured my interest. That gem in the flesh was my co-worker Karen. Karen was the epitome of what I desired to be as a vegan. Instead of berating me for my choices, she emailed me a few links and recommended that I check them out. The aura around her was ecstatically pleasing. I felt compelled to do more research after speaking with her. Although I didn't consider veganism until months later when my health began to decline, had I felt belittled or dull-witted by her reaction to my lifestyle, I may have rebelled against it.

Being labeled the nice vegan once I became known for my lifestyle wasn't too shocking to me. I appreciate the label, but I'm disappointed that we continue to demonstrate a behavior that evolved from a feud with omnivores, to a squabble within the vegan community on who's considered a true vegan. Despite personal aspirations to transition, we should still welcome and support people who actually eat a vegan diet. It's the support from our communities that allowed us to get this far and to make this much progress.

The most prominent concern within our communities is bullying. Bullying has become a serious issue over the years especially since social media has grown. Attacking someone for failing to meet every expectation is an act of insanity. Everyone is responsible for their own actions and a lot of nonprofit animal rights organizations share the blame for encouraging this nonsensical behavior. Whatever vision you have to make a change in this world should always be done in an effective peaceful manner. It doesn't appear the vegan community has mastered this on an optimal level. Let's discuss the history and take a look at the facts.

Donald Watson who started as a member of the UK Vegetarian Society, later founded The Vegan Society in 1945. He had a strong passion to influence people to change their relationship with food, and fortunate enough for him, the Vegetarian Society was a platform for him to do that. He was preeminently kind, welcoming, and truly concerned for human health which led to his growing views for the future of dieting. Watson began to share his ideas with fellow members who, in turn, supported his innovative ideas and joined his movement. His passion became stronger when he noticed the reception from his followers as he began to implement a new path to dieting. His plan was to take the vegetarian diet to the next level by eliminating all animal products. Gaining confidence and outpouring support from fellow members, Watson knew the time had come for him to take action. He proposed his ideas to The Vegetarian Society's board in hopes of using their platform to disseminate his message. Captivated by his readiness to make a difference, the non-dairy group gained access to use the Vegetarian Messenger to reach a larger audience.

The first letter published in 1944 by Watson's new group captured public attention. The recognition prompted the group to decide on a name for their new style of dieting that would separate them from the vegetarian name. The group decided to move forward with the name *Vegan* to make it unique, but similar to the name people were already accustomed to. Watson's goal was to attract people to become health-conscious individuals and to refrain from consuming animal products. Although veganism did not have a society of its own at the time, their first newsletter revealed pertinent information in regard to their plans for the future.

Below are three points I'd like to make from Watson's first newsletter in 1944:

1.) Watson's early letters were publicized on the Vegetarian Messenger. The groups worked together and had a mutual respect for each other's approach. When deciding on a name for their non-dairy vegetarian group, the term vegan was meticulously chosen as an effort to avoid anything that appeared unwelcoming. He believed the term *non-dairy* was restrictive, negative, and unattractive to their new approach to dieting. He wanted to have the same ethical standard as The Vegetarian Society with the absence of dairy. He described veganism as a diet and made few suggestions about lifestyle changes. Animal rights activists were not a part of the vegan movement at that time and did not play a role in the implementation process to influence others to consider dietary changes.

2.) Watson knew the controversy that would come from creating a new dietary approach. He made the following statement in an attempt to avoid potential misunderstandings:

> "In any case, there need to be no animosity between ourselves and the 'lactos'. We all accept that lacto-vegetarianism has a well-appointed place in the dietary evolution, and for this reason several of us spend a great deal of our time working for the lacto-vegetarian cause."

3.) While addressing dietary concerns in his newsletter, Watson stated something that stood out to me. In his rebuttal on the misconceptions of a plant-only diet, he mentioned that, from his knowledge, every member of their group was no longer consuming animal products for humanitarian reasons (not animal rights). I thought this was interesting since nowadays people often associate veganism with animal rights only. Some vegans even encounter dissociation by other vegans for not converting for the purpose of animal rights. This shows how time has changed since the inception of veganism since there were a variety of reasons (excluding animal rights) to transition to a vegan diet. The only requirement at that time was to remove all animal products from your diet. If you were eating a plant-only diet, then you were considered vegan.

Donald Watson's first newsletter, Nov. 1944

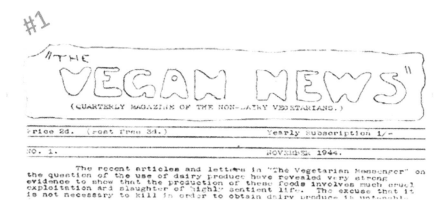

In 1945, the new vegan non-dairy vegetarian group committee met for the first time in London to start their organization called The Vegan Society. In conclusion of the committee meeting, a manifesto was published by Watson:

> "The Aims of The Vegan Society are: **1.)** To advocate that man's food should be derived from fruits, nuts, vegetables, grains, and other wholesome non-animal products and that it should exclude flesh, fish, fowl, eggs, honey, animals' milk, butter, and cheese. **2.)** To encourage the manufacture, and use of alternatives to animal commodities."

As we can see, the manifesto only encouraged people to refrain from using animal commodities. The history as we know it today does not align with what actually occurred in early years. The historical timeline may not seem relevant but knowing the intentions of the founders debunks a lot of misconceptions. Watson started the society in the United Kingdom. As the society aged, the UK Vegan Society misreported a few historical events for many years. These events are relevant to what the organization represented prior to the influence of animal activists. I don't believe any actions taken by the society were intentional; however, the information provided for public knowledge should be accurate and corrected. In 1962, for example, co-founder Elisie Shrigley inadvertently (I'm presuming), proclaimed The Vegan Society was founded in November 1944. Although the society was founded in 1945, and this may seem irrelevant, it shows how the society continues to overlook the history to focus on today's organizational goals to promote the new vegan identity created by animal activists.

The assertion by Elisie Shrigley that the society was founded in 1944 in the spring 1962 issue:

> The first meeting of 8 non-dairy vegetarians to choose a name and found the Society was in November, 1944, at the Attic Club in Holborn. It was a Sunday, with sunshine and blue sky, an auspicious day for the birth of an idealistic movement. From a long list of suggestions the word Vegan was chosen. This name is now known all over the world. It has appeared in medical, scientific and other journals, in the daily press, and on the B.B.C.

The only action that took place in 1944 was the invention of the word *Vegan* and Walton's first newsletter. This is just one of the few misleading statements that play a vital role in the constant battles we see within the vegan community today. Everyone claims to know the facts, even when some information is misreported.

During Watson's days as a member of the Vegetarian Society, he briefly expressed his concerns for the mistreatment of our animals in slaughter-houses. He was highly compassionate toward animals and encouraged members who were interested to consider removing animal commodities in addition to making dietary changes. His intentions were never to promote changes that extended outside of the vegan diet, but to encourage the idea for those who were interested in a lifestyle change. The position he adopted was no different than the Vegetarian Society's objective to promote healthier dietary choices. As with vegetarianism, everything beyond an individual's diet was at the members' discretion. He had no desire to force his personal views on members or to form a cult-like society that was violent and unkind.

There was a great amount of investment placed into the vision that welcomed people who were interested in abiding by the strict diet while advocating for the movement. The vision seemed clear, but uncertainty from any part of leadership enables anyone to come in and force an identity on it. The requirements were already written and stated, so the emphasis placed on what was simply encouraged was the beginning of a new vegan identity.

Watson wasn't new to the violence displayed by animal activists. He advocated for the animals as well, but he did not agree with how things were being handled in an effort to bring recognition to the mistreatment of animals. He knew veganism would catch the attention of many animal activists, which he welcomed, but he also knew the labels they carried. He wanted to make his intentions clear to the world on what the vegan movement represented. He specifically advised *"In any case, there need be no animosity between ourselves and the 'lactos'."* Everyone holds opinions about how things should function, but the truth is that veganism at that time was nothing more than a vegetarian diet with the absence of dairy products. He wanted to be a better representation of a lifestyle that promoted a safe environment, healthy living, and an ideal relationship between animals and humans.

Excerpt from Watson's first newsletter:

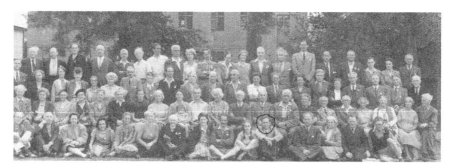

Donald Watson (1947) IVU (International Vegetarian Union) – World Vegetarian Congress

From 1945 to 1946, Watson and his founders were still in limbo about how they wanted to function as an organization. I believe there was a lot of pressure in keeping and recruiting members who were receptive to the changes they were implementing. In spring of 1947, Fay K. Henderson, UK Vegan Society secretary, published a list of commandments called *The Vegan Way of Life*.

"The Vegan Society has been formed to coordinate and assist these pioneers in their efforts, it has a threefold aim:

1. To advocate that man's food should be derived from fruits, nuts, vegetables, grains and other wholesome non-animal products, and that it should exclude flesh, fish, fowl, eggs, honey, animals' milk, butter and cheese;

2. To encourage the production and use of alternatives to animal commodities"

THE
VEGAN
SOCIETY

ADVOCATES
that mans food should be derived from nuts, fruits, vegetables and grains.
ENCOURAGES
the use of alternatives to all products of animal origin.
DETAILS FROM THE SECRETARY
RYDAL LODGE, AMBLESIDE, WESTMORLAND

This was also advised in the manifesto that was published after the committee meeting in 1945. During the time of this publication, there had to be an internal conflict arising because by the next annual meeting that following year (1948), Watson retired. I'm sure this came as a surprise for many considering the fact it was still a fairly new society. There were rumors of him being bullied by animal rights extremists to make changes he did not agree with by members of the organization. There were also rumors that the UK Vegetarian Society was pressured a few times as well but refused. It was known that the UK Vegetarian Society was not making any changes after officially establishing their set of rules and requirements. The Vegan Society was not as confident with their approach since changes for them were recurring.

A few noteworthy things happened upon Watson's retirement in 1948:

1) Leslie J. Cross, animal rights activists (referred to as an extremist) and member of Vegan Society since 1946, was elected as a board member.
2) Honey was banned from the vegan diet for the first time.
3) Watson was presented with a permanent honorary award that meant he was acknowledged for the role he played within the organization.

It wasn't long after Watson stepped down that the Society took a turn for the worse. Things began to change quickly, due in part to the addition of many other animal rights extremists who played a major role in corrupting The Vegan Society's reputation.

Leslie J. Cross turned out to be a narcissist. His position as a board member gave him leverage in the decision-making process that impacted the future of the society. He didn't join the UK Vegan Society to abide by their rules; he joined to gain control over the organization to change it to reflect his beliefs. Less than a year after becoming a board member, Cross meticulously planned his approach to put his ideas and beliefs on the forefront in hopes of shifting the focus. The summer of 1949 newsletter changed everything for members of the society. Cross took a rather smart move in his approach by announcing how the society failed to decide on a clear definition for veganism. He was so wrapped up in his personal agenda that he carried on, further advising that previous attempts to define veganism was premature since the society was still finding its way.

IN SEARCH OF VEGANISM—1.

By Leslie J. Cross

CLEARING THE GROUND

The present stage in the development of The Vegan Society is characterized by a centering of attention upon the implications of the question, " What is veganism ? "

. There is more—much more—behind this disarmingly simple query than at first appears. To begin with, we have to clear our minds of certain assumptions ; to realise, for example, that when, we say, " Veganism is this, or that," what we are really saying is; " My idea of veganism is this, or that." For there is nothing in the constitution of The Vegan Society which states what veganism is.

The fact that the Society has reached its present position without having defined in any precise way the light it attempts to reflect need not disturb us. There were good, if perhaps unrecognised, reasons why definition should not be attempted until the Society reached a certain point along its road. What, however,

What remained clear is that Watson had already established a solid following during his involvement with the Society. He stated in multiple newsletters what the requirements were and what was simply encouraged. The Society gained its popularity on those facts. Cross wanted to promote an entire lifestyle rather than the diet that caught most members' attention from the beginning. It was no different than what the Vegetarian Society was promoting in regards to dietary changes. Yes, both organizations have their own core values, but none that excluded any members who did not change anything beyond their diet. Cross morphed the society into something that was distasteful, unwelcoming, and controversial.

Cross's whole objective was to redefine veganism to be limited to animal rights; this definition ended up excluding more than half of the current members. He didn't want to give Watson the credit for the success of the society. He went as far as insinuating that Watson stole his idea and he was really the mastermind behind the movement. No one fed into his accusations, but it does make you wonder how someone could corrupt such an empowering movement single-handedly.

A disastrous outcome seemed to occur every year in the early years of The Vegan Society's annual meetings. Board members, along with members of the organization, would attend these meetings to give their input on organizational restructuring. Cross decided to take advantage of his first annual meeting as a board member by ensuring a few of his animal rights activist friends and supporters were present to propose his argument on redefining veganism and changing the requirements. He gained enough votes to get his proposal passed.

Cross managed to gain full control over The Vegan Society that day. Under the new regulations, the below occurred:

- Watson was robbed of his lifetime honorary role in the organization as a VP
- All the other honorary non-active lifetime vice presidents were replaced
- Cross was promoted to Executive Vice President
- More than half of the board members who came in under Watson were replaced
- The Vegan newsletter editor resigned (Watson supporter)

And there you have it. In just one day and with a little manipulation, Cross managed to take over an entire organization by replacing every member who played a key role in building the vegan name and reputation. Every aspect of the organization (other than its name) was changed and transformed into a cult-like organization. Cross didn't show any form of homage to the founders or original committee members who brought the attention and success to The Vegan Society.

The foundation built by these organizations is in support of animal rights but also in support of helping people create a sustainable diet and lifestyle. Veganism and vegetarianism are both sustainable lifestyles, but a lot of people do not have the determination and commitment required to live this way. Vegetarianism is a great alternative to build confidence to one day transition to a vegan diet. Cross promoted a lifestyle that disregarded the importance of human health. His vision was primarily focused on the importance of nonhuman lives and how humans should avoid harming animals at all cost. The cost includes compromising their health because of the lack of information and attention placed on a healthy sustainable vegan diet.

Followers were able to see what Cross really stood for because of his transparency. When Cross took over, the focal point shifted and resulted in over 450 active paying members to become frustrated to the point of canceling their membership. No one was interested in joining, so The Vegan Society had little to no hope in staying afloat. After six long years (1950-1956) of bringing the organization down to its last days, Cross decided to resign. His resignation had to be the best thing that ever happened for the vegan movement.

There are three driving forces that will always be the lifeline of The Vegan Society. In fact, these three forces are what led the society to a season of prosperity:

1.) Human Health
2.) Environmental Health
3.) Animal Welfare

A lifestyle with little purpose is no service to the community. It's quite evident that the three forces (human health, environmental health, and animal welfare) mesh together. One of these forces cannot thrive without the other. If health is of paramount importance to you, then protecting our environment and closing slaughter-houses automatically becomes a part of your agenda. That applies to the other forces as well. Let's put this in perspective, if someone decides to transition to help protect our environment, isn't that also pushing the agenda to end animal cruelty since animal agriculture is the culprit for increasing the level of carbon dioxide contributing to global warming?

Let's take this perspective a little further; if you're an animal activist consuming mainly ultra-processed foods, wouldn't it be safe to say you're not a true vegan since human health was initially the primary focus? Watson described vegan foods as *wholesome* non-animal products. Ultra-processed foods have many ingredients that are not categorized as wholesome foods. Regardless of what someone struggles with outside their diet does not warrant isolation or judgment. No one should feel ostracized because their diet alone isn't enough to be a part of the movement. Bullying is always unacceptable. Veganism should be a movement for unity and peace. If one chooses to promote health or take environmental responsibility as opposed to shifting their concerns towards animal rights, then let them play that vital role within the community. The ultimate goal is to attract people to veganism by promoting the three forces, not to push people away.

Authority Figures

The changes in authority figures over the years and their difference in views created an opportunity for members to feel entitled to choose what constitution they would follow. Some authority figures eventually returned to the original proposal that aligned with Watson's approach pertaining to eating a healthy plant-only diet. Other authority figures promoted Cross's approach claiming it evolved from a diet to a lifestyle that strictly prohibited members from using anything that contain animal products (makeup, soap, clothing, etc.). Sadly, members began to create their own extreme rules such as not supporting organizations that sell animal products even if it's supporting their cruelty-free line/products. Things started changing exponentially and members were becoming more segregated because of their beliefs and lifestyle.

Cross's departure was due to health complications, but the damage he'd done remained. During the 1950s, The Vegan Society treasurer showed records of more than 80 cancellations, with little to no new memberships. These events combined produced a financial loss.

During this time of turmoil, the remaining board members along with the new newsletter editor, John Heron, decided to save the society. John was not a great fit for his position considering his lack of knowledge on veganism. He promoted the idea of segregating people based on their beliefs. Not only was he a complete novice to veganism, but he was clueless on what attracted members to the society in the first place. After seeing how many people were eating a vegan diet for health purposes, especially those in the United States, Heron felt compelled to advise that *health-based vegans* were not vegans at all but hygienists. He alluded that some were transitioning for religious purposes and should not identify themselves as vegans at all. His approach was to find labels to describe health vegans and spiritual vegans, thus insinuating that they were not true to the vegan lifestyle. This was one of the primary reasons why vegans and animal activists today have grown to promote segregation within the community.

I can't begin to describe the foolishness of it all. Everyone today is confused, no one cares to learn the history, and no one who held a position within the society cared enough to consult their predecessors to learn from their mistakes. The Vegan Society was merely an idea waiting on an identity. Anytime doubt is in the equation, the result is like a feather in the air – it will go wherever the wind blows.

The global rise of veganism over the years wasn't because of the promotion of animal rights. The rise was a result of promoting a healthy diet that doesn't harm our animals or environment. The vast majority of vegans were in it for health purposes. When health was nearly the only topic of discussion, new membership was on the rise; when it began to shift to primarily animal rights, hardly anyone was joining and membership cancellation was at an all-time high.

Emotional Impact

We are emotional creatures who respond emotionally to the things that we are passionate about. Sharing the same moral compass as the Vegetarian Society, you'd think unity would be the society's strongest asset within our communities. Instead, we all have different passions so our emotional responses to the issues we face are different.

Health advocates are not rebellions who signed a petition to officially disregard animal welfare. It's an act of putting human health first. Changing your diet can be extremely difficult when you're used to eating meat and dairy all your life. People who are doing it for health purposes are challenging themselves, so their fight is waged internally. They are not at war with the outside world or those who choose not to embark on the vegan journey. They are humble and rarely speak on their diet or engage in any political debates on the lifestyle.

On the other hand, environmentalists are very passionate people. Their diet is rarely the topic of discussion; however, they are vocal about their concerns about how animal agriculture is harming our environment. They are sometimes aggressive in their approach only because they are such passionate people, but it's harmless. Every aspect of their lives is about environmental sustainability and reducing unnecessary waste. Although they are passionate, they are not bullies. They do not attack you based on your lifestyle or way of living. They are very welcoming; if you're interested, consider joining the "Go Green" movement.

Lastly, animal rights activists are like the trouble child in the vegan community. They are the reason vegans were labeled extremists. They are very aggressive and defensive in their approach. They are seeking nothing more than pure perfection from those interested in the animal rights movement. A few of them are not aggressive, violent, or open for debates like the vast majority; however, once engaged, you can expect them to express themselves without filter. They rarely speak on the adverse impact meat has on our environment and overall health. Some have no limitation on their actions against those who challenge their views. They rarely show concern for human health or are cautious of the food they eat. As long as their meals don't include animal products, they are satisfied enough. Bullying has become a reputation of theirs towards people who do not share the same values and beliefs. They are primarily the reason why plant-only eaters do not claim to be vegan. Although this is true for most animal activist, I want to be clear that this does not apply to all.

We need passionate people to speak out on these issues. We should also speak out on bullying and identify this behavior and negative energy as it permeates our communities. Bullying prevents a positive outcome in any situation; it does not get results.

As we progress and reach a new level of success, we also reach a new level of ignorance. It certainly seems we gravitate towards supporting the force that best aligns with our values and beliefs. This could only happen by acknowledging how we've become so divided. Each member brings a unique aspect to the community that allows us to thrive in areas that were once unachievable. Working together to reach a common goal will allow us to form a more cohesive unity. Instead of breaking our people down, let's educate and encourage them to take a stand with us. If they are not interested in changing every aspect of their lives, applaud them for their efforts. We need to be a bit more merciful toward those who have not reached our level of veganism. It's a fight within us all. The reality now is that food and animal commodities have graduated from simple *luxuries* to full-blown habits and addictions that are not easy to break.

Chapter 3

Plant-Based Diet v. Plant-Only Diet

"It is easier to change a man's religion than to change his diet."

~ Margaret Mead

Incorporating new healthy habits to protect your health is admirable. The lifestyle you adopt could never downplay your efforts to make a change. Keeping that in mind, let's discuss each label and its unique approach to dieting. A plant-based diet and a vegan diet are often used interchangeably, but they refer to two very different lifestyles. Event organizers in support of veganism commonly advertise events using both labels, but the food options only align with a vegan diet. Not that anyone attending would expect to see animal products on the menu; it's the confusion surrounding the labels. A plant-based diet has its own set of restrictions that minimize the use of processed foods. This type of diet consists of foods primarily derived from plants. Foods that fall within the plant category are fruits, vegetables, legumes, whole grains, nuts, and seeds.

A plant-based diet is not an alternative label for vegan. Minimizing processed foods is only one part of it. The lifestyle is much like a starter kit for a healthier way of living. It's not a diet that supports elimination, but minimization. The elimination of animal products in a plant-based diet is at the dieter's discretion. Meat and dairy are still optional and can be included in daily meals. A plant-based diet offers more flexibility. It's also a frequently used term to avoid the moral and ethical standard that comes with the vegan name. Because of the inherent flexibility, most people find this to be an ideal approach to sustaining a healthy lifestyle.

The Vegan Way

Veganism demands a better environment for all living things. Sometimes too demanding that the lifestyle seems to support division rather than inclusion, but that's never the case. Its purpose serves a higher meaning that sends shock waves through our communities. Feeling ostracized is a normal emotion when you're surviving on the other side. Hanging out with a group of vegans could make you feel out of place or judged. Sometimes that is the case, but pace yourself and move at your own speed. You don't have to show your undying love for animals if that's not what you're in it for. If you're in it for your health, then scream that at the top of your lungs. Watson was neutral and wasn't too focused on either. Overall health for all living things was his goal. Fighting with our inner urges is one thing, but we want nothing more than to thrive as healthy human beings. Non-humans have the right to do the same and thrive in their natural habitat. If I had to define the movement, it's a solution for human and non-human lives to escape this vicious cycle of toxic living.

The foundation of The Vegan Society that brought in financial support was built on the need for healthier alternatives. Both health and animal rights are of equal importance in the vegan fight. Because veganism parallels perfectly with other aspects of healthy living, it makes it undeniably fitting for mankind.

The beginnings of veganism were developed in the United Kingdom. By the time the movement migrated to the United States, it was surrounded by a health cautious buzz. As Americans, we were focused on ourselves before we acknowledged how veganism benefited everything else. We shouldn't have to choose what holds the most weight in the vegan movement anyway, since we're all in this together. Let's enjoy everything it has to offer. We're so anxious to call out the imperfections of our brothers and sisters that we don't realize the adverse effects it has on our overall growth. We live in a society where we will criticize people based on their actions and beliefs before we extend a helping hand. Let's be a helping hand for a world that needs us.

A Plant-Based Diet Is NOT a Plant-Only Diet

A plant-based diet and a plant-only diet are very similar. They consist primarily of whole foods; hence little to no processed foods, and both offer an ideal option for people who are struggling with health issues. Plant-only is a term rarely used and holds the most benefits. It was a term used for many years prior to my existence. When I would meticulously read through Watson's early newsletters, I noticed he compared veganism to a plant-only diet. It stood out to me because it highlighted his vision for nature and its species. When Watson left the organization, veganism was no longer a plant-only diet that supported healthy living. It became a cruelty-free diet welcoming a wide range of processed foods.

The cruelty-free name came about after the activists for animal liberation gained control over the organization. This is what created the rise in using plant-based as a vegan term. People began to opt for a healthier way of living while escaping the animal rights madness. It was a commonly used term that was forced on people who did not live up to the vegan standard. As often as the term plant-based is used, people rarely eat a plant-based diet. It's just another term that offers mental comfort and flexibility.

Katherine D. McManus, MS, RD, LDN (2018) posted on the Harvard Health blog an inspirational plant-based guide, and a few plant-based meals to get you started.[10] For breakfast, she advised a typical meal would be scrambled eggs with veggies wrapped in a whole-wheat tortilla. She proceeded with a lunch recommendation which was a vegetarian pizza with mozzarella cheese on top. Plant-based meals recommended by most healthcare professionals (dietitians and nutritionists) include meat and dairy products, just a smaller portion.

There is nothing wrong with supporting a plant-based diet even if you're not on one. If a cruelty –free lifestyle is the message you want to send to your audience, then you may want to refrain from using plant-based as a way to describe your lifestyle. Some may argue that the definition states *"minimize or eliminate meat,"* however, the option is still open for the dieter to make the decision on what they'd like to do. Whatever lifestyle you choose to live or promote, just ensure it's something you stand by with certainty. If your passion is to inspire the world to use plants as a source of food, then promoting a plant-based diet could be misleading to your audience.

Plant-Only Diet v. Cruelty-Free Diet (Vegan)

When the movement began, there was no talk about processed foods or finding meat-like alternatives. As I mentioned earlier, Watson promoted a health-driven diet that was best described as a plant-only diet. There were specific food groups stated and published to describe the upcoming dietary movement which consisted of fruits, veggies, grains, nuts, and seeds. The food groups were listed by the founders to

---

[10] Katherine D. McManus, MS, RD, LDN, *What is a plant-based diet and why should you try it?* (Harvard Health Publishing, 2018), url https://www.health.harvard.edu/blog/what-is-a-plant-based-diet-and-why-should-you-try-it-2018092614760

set the trajectory of the movement. Human health was of great importance in the duration of Watson's involvement with the society, and the statements made by him and his team reflected it. As veganism evolved under different leaderships, the objective shifted. Many vegans today consume a large amount of highly processed foods because human health is no longer the foundation of the movement. Protecting our animals is nothing short of important, but it's ignorant to challenge ourselves to eliminate animal products and conquer all just to excuse the most important threat to our body, which is ultra-processed food.

I know there's this seemingly innocuous question lingering in the air with an attempt to confirm that a plant-only diet (often mistaken as a plant-based diet), is the same as a cruelty-free diet (vegan diet). A plant-only diet embraces nature and encourages that followers eat living foods that nourish the body while excluding all animal products. A plant-based diet is an attempt to do the same, but it doesn't quite meet the standard since a small portion of animal products are acceptable. A cruelty-free diet is self-explanatory: anything that doesn't include animal products is acceptable. The confusion arises when people presume a cruelty-free diet is a healthy diet because animal products are the problem. What makes your diet unhealthy is not meat alone. Simple carbs and unhealthy fats are contributing factors in damaging our health. The chemicals the meat companies place in our food to make them larger, more colorful, and longer lasting, damage our health as well. Also, eating too much or too little of anything can lead to health complications. The list could go on, but the point is that meat is not the culprit of an overall unhealthy diet. Veganism has taken on its own identity over the years, which at this point could only be defined as a cruelty-free diet. Veganism today no longer aligns with a plant-only diet.

The label we gravitate to is not what's important. The most important aspect of changing your diet is the nourishment the food provides. Your choice of food must complement your body's daily needs. Every source of protein, fats, and carbs are not the healthiest, which is why it's crucial that we listen to our body's needs. If you're new to a healthy way of living, the best way to start is educating yourself on basic whole foods and why they're the best foods to consume. Also, take the time to learn more about superfoods, vitamins, minerals, and antioxidants. This information will provide you with more understanding about what foods to choose and the best way to consume them (e.g., raw/juiced or cooked). I know this may sound crazy, but as a novice, it can be challenging to make a change with little to no insight about what to do or where to start. The average person who eats a thoughtless diet probably only knows the basics from what was taught in school. They couldn't readily explain why fruits and vegetables (whole foods) are healthy; all they know is that certain foods are said to be healthy and the unenlightened cycle continues.

As curious as I was about this being the case with most people, I decided to test my theory prior to writing this book. I met a woman in her mid-20s who finally decided to learn more about healthy living by changing her diet. After four months of being vegan, I asked her if she could name five minerals. As I expected, she couldn't. Then, I asked her if she had ever heard of iron, sodium, potassium, calcium, or zinc, and she instantly felt insulted. She only felt insulted because she couldn't believe that I thought she had never heard of potassium, calcium, iron, etc., but in fact I was confirming my theory, but also bringing light to the fact that you can't start a new dietary lifestyle without practicing some form of self-education. Don't get me wrong, you can be clueless on these things and hire a nutritionist/dietitian to educate you. Realistically, who has the money or time? Even with hiring a dietitian or nutritionist, their primary job function is to educate you. This goes back to what I mentioned in chapter two about relying on others to tell us what's healthy and what isn't. We must research and make decisions based on what we know and learn, not what we hear from a supposed subject-matter expert.

Is a Plant-Based Diet Healthy?

A plant-based diet has its health benefits, but portion size plays a significant role in how the body responds to it. Fruit sugar, complex carbs, and olive oil are healthy, but an excessive amount can lead to unwanted weight gain and health complications. Too much of anything can lead to a series of health challenges, especially unwanted weight gain from eating more calories than the body burns in a day. Arguing that an unhealthy plant-based diet is when you incorporate highly processed foods, such as cookies, cakes, ice cream, etc. is describing a lifestyle that doesn't fit. A plant-based diet is derived from plants and minimally processed foods. Cookies, cakes, and ice cream do not fit into the unhealthy plant-based category since it was never included from start. What's strange about how things have transpired over the years is hearing people label themselves as plant-based eaters while actually eating a cruelty-free diet. The contradiction is plant-based eaters will incorporate a great amount of processed foods in their plant-based diet but argue that they converted for health purposes. Promoting healthy living is a wonderful thing, but to actually live it is even better.

Did you know that a meat eater who consumes primarily whole foods lives an overall healthier life than vegans who consume primarily processed food? As much as vegans promote healthy living, some eat more processed food than meat eaters. People who claim plant-based aren't actually eating a plant-based diet, but a cruelty-free diet. Some are eating a plant-only diet, but the majority of the people who are, don't realize it because of their lack of knowledge.

We are in a time where everyone tries to be technical about everything. Vegans are arguing with vegans about who's the real vegan; vegetarians are frustrated with vegans for their constant attacks on the misrepresentation of a cruelty-free lifestyle, and plant-based/plant-only eaters are so adamant about breaking free from all the judgment that they often lose sight of what they are truly promoting. Meanwhile, most companies that sponsor events such as the Vegan Fest welcome everyone. These companies cater to vegans and non-vegans daily and do not discriminate at the doors of these events to weed out those who don't meet the vegan standard. They uplift people to consider transitioning. We created this aggressive approach because of our own passion for the lifestyle.

The Abandon Plant-Only Diet

You'll rarely hear the term plant-only, but it's real and the closest thing to a raw vegan diet. It's actually more restrictive than a vegan diet. In the mist of all the chaos that comes with the different labels, a plant-based label is the most accepted. It allows a person to eliminate all animal products from their diet while gaining acceptance by the society that finds the vegan movement eccentric and tyrannical.

The plant-based diet is interesting as it specifically caters to both vegans and meat eaters. These minor tweaks in the diet allow two very different lifestyles to come together by formulating the healthiest version of each dietary preference by limiting access to processed foods. We all know that people are not too fond of restrictions, especially when it comes to their diet and abiding by a strict set of dietary rules. It is not something they set out to do.

It is becoming more common to seek other practices that improve different areas of life. More people are finding natural alternatives for skin care, hair care, oral care, etc. that are healthy and effective. Eastern medicine is being practiced more and appears to be increasing. It's not uncommon for people to start making lifestyle changes and building new healthy habits beyond their diet. A plant-only diet, whether raw or cooked, usually is the end goal for people who want to make adjustments that focus on them entirely. It may not be a commonly used term, but people are using their food as medicine and have dedicated their lives to living on a plant-only diet. Not just for the sake of healthy living, but for environmental purposes since it directly affects the air we breathe and the food we eat.

When I became ill, I started my journey on a raw, plant-only diet. I didn't identify it as a raw vegan diet. Honestly, I didn't label myself at all because the only desire I had was to improve my health. The animal rights movement was certainly the last thing on my mind. Now that I'm more knowledgeable on the history and the purpose of veganism and other dietary lifestyles, I realize labels are nothing more than a forced identity.

Social Influence

Society has an unwavering influence on how people think and behave. It's easier to attach labels on others now that social media is the modus operandi for communicating with the outside world. The moral standard is highly valued and can be the subject of a debate when certain actions don't align. These actions are usually associated with the use of animal commodities. This has always been known to happen and having access to a larger group of people on social sites such as Facebook and Twitter, made it easier to target people who would have otherwise been unreachable. This isn't to single out a group of people, but who can we blame? Where does the change begin? We could blame the animal activists or each individual for their role in the attacks, but why should we blame anyone other than ourselves? The change starts with us being better advocates for what we stand for. The organizations that embrace the movement have to stand for what's right and stop making excuses for the behavior of their members. We all are frustrated and annoyed with the ignorance, but it's never an excuse to antagonize or attack people out of anger.

There are organizations that speak out on their nonviolent movement, but when an incident occurs with one of their members, they sometimes find a way to make it acceptable. The circumstances surrounding their position are understandable; however, while acting as a leader of a movement, there should be a set of core values that are more important. We have to stand for all human and non-human lives. Bullying isn't something that only happens among our children/youth. Having an outlet or a source for validation is important to people who are vulnerable and seeking acceptance. How we treat them is what they will remember us for.

Anyone has the ability to share their thoughts about your decisions whenever they want. Bullying isn't always carried out by people we know; most times, it's from complete strangers who are passionately expressing their beliefs. Because there is no way to truly mitigate cyber bullying, it's important for us to stand collectively and show our disapproval.

Animal Activist Defense

Animal activists have held protests and supporting events prior to The Vegan Society, even years before Watson came along. As the founder, Watson experienced the cruel mistreatment of being ostracized as well. There is no exemption from unfair treatment when something is said or done that goes against the standard. You didn't have to know Watson personally or experience him during his vegan journey to know what type of leader he wanted to be. His written words proved he was more than a leader, but someone who showed love and gratitude to those that supported him and his ideas along his journey.

Sarah Gate's article in The Independent newspaper, called *"Calling vegans 'extremists' leads to violence – what we really want is to talk,"* discusses how reckless it is to refer to vegans as extremists since it suggests that vegans condone violence. The headline was confusing to me because calling someone an extremist doesn't lead to violence. Their reaction to being called an extremist does. As she continued in her defense for the animal rights community, she failed to acknowledge why the term extremist surfaced in the first place. I'm a vegan and even I know why that term surfaced. Our failure to acknowledge why things are the way they are, creates a roadblock between us and the people we'd like to influence. The first step in resolving any problem is acknowledging your faults to fix the part you have control over. Bringing awareness to anyone else's faults in a situation is like throwing water on a grease fire.

The example Gate used to support the misconception she believed to be unfair is the Alison Waugh (animal farmer) incident with BBC News. Apparently, Waugh told BBC News she received death threats from animal activists because of her profession. When other farmers heard Waugh's story, they began sharing similar encounters of receiving death threats. The entire incident led to a public frenzy. Because of the attention Waugh received from her interview with BBC news, she recanted her statement, stating that she had never received death threats from anyone. I personally found this disheartening and inconsiderate to the voices of many other farmers who actually experienced this and gained the courage to speak out. This incident is something that makes it harder for animal activists and farmers to have their voices heard.

Gate decided to promote the idea that farmers are willing to lie to perpetuate what she believes to be a misconception, but things like this occur frequently. Instead of acknowledging what could have been done differently, Gate insinuated that animal activists were the victims. Her entire article disregarded the history. The blame was placed on farmers for being the cause of most escalated situations. Gate seemed to be on the side of fostering camaraderie, but her perspective of what's happening in the world of non-human rights was primarily based on her personal experiences with people within her social circle.

There is no excuse for animal activists or farmers to respond with violence. The reputation of animal activists doesn't encourage farmers or companies in the meat and dairy industry to be less defensive during their interactions. In years prior to veganism, animal activists were violent and aggressive in their approach. In fact, they were labeled extremists because of their behavior. I agree that we need people to protest to bring awareness to the mistreatment of our animals and how it affects our health and environment, but how we deliver our message is just as important as getting our message across.

I do not condone any violent or aggressive behavior, so this is not an attempt to take sides. I will always stand by our environment and animals until the death of me. I just experienced life on both sides of the fence and can empathize with all parties. As vegans, we are comfortable protesting and fighting for what's right because we know how life is without fulfilling our agenda to abolish all forms of animal use. We are still able to work and provide for our families and live life as we know it.

Farmers, on the other hand, have more to lose in this fight. They are in that line of business to provide for their families and a majority of them are not in the business by choice necessarily, but by habit and what was handed down to them from generation to generation. In most cases, it's all they know. What we are doing is threatening to end life as they know it. To them, we are more than just people who are protesting; we are a major threat to their livelihood, and our approach is even more threatening when we insinuate that protecting our animals is more important than their livelihood. Everything has to be taken into consideration, and we need to remember that they are fighting for what they know as normalcy.

I expect nothing less than a brutal attack for considering non-vegan concerns. Some vegans would consider their feelings to be irrelevant since what we are doing is for the greater good. If their feelings and concerns don't matter, why are we protesting? You have to ask these questions before making a hasty decision to attack anyone who tries to empathize with farmers. What we need to understand is that it's ok to care about non-vegan lives. Caring won't make you any less of a vegan and definitely doesn't make you a traitor. This is the reason why The Vegan Society is operating in a way that caters to the feelings of only vegans as opposed to taking a stand when horrible things are happening in the name of veganism. This has to stop at some point. As I mentioned in Chapter 2, The Vegetarian Society refused to allow animal activists to step in and disrupt the peaceful encouraging lifestyle they worked so hard to create.

As a person who previously couldn't live without consuming animal products, I can empathize with people who are not interested in veganism because I was that person once. It's imperative to consider the following when approaching someone who has never experienced life without meat:

- Avoid entering into someone's personal space
- Avoid referring to their lifestyle as a luxury, but as an addiction or a paying job to feed their family
- Avoid discussing a cruelty-free diet in restaurants or during meals
- Avoid facial expressions that shows disgust or criticism
- Avoid aggressive behavior

Try the below for the most effective approach:

- One-on-one interaction
- Plan ahead in a receptive atmosphere
- Propose a solution for a career change, food alternatives, etc.
- When discussing these issues, ask for approval to share your concerns
- If you sense things are getting out of control, end the protest
- Encourage feedback from your listeners
- Show appreciation to your listeners

The purpose of protesting is to object to the mistreatment of non-human lives. It's to encourage people to reconsider their choices while taking into consideration what's at stake. What's better than creating a marketing strategy to attract people to the vegan lifestyle versus raising hostility in everyone? The latter would produce no results and no solution, just a community full of angry people.

I enjoy everything about nature and the idea of our animals embracing life in their natural habitat. I have no desire to influence farmers or meat eaters to continue the cycle of killing our animals while damaging our environment and our health. From personal experience, when things wouldn't go as I intended, I'd yell and scream and sometimes attack the person who challenged me. Every time I did that, I realized I made the situation worse for myself. I made it difficult to achieve my goals. I don't want our behavior to prevent us from reaching our milestones. Being less reactive is a small change that can lead to phenomenal results.

In Conclusion (Part 1) . . .

Part 1 of this book covers the importance of dieting, transitioning, social influence, and the fight we are facing in the vegan community.

Transitioning to veganism can be a challenging process, but being clear on your purpose for embarking on the vegan journey makes the fight worth it. Discovering your inner passion for veganism and exploring the different diets will help ensure a smooth transition. Your passion does not have to be confined to animal rights. Any force that enables you to give your best (Environmental Health, Human Health, or Animal Welfare) is what matters. If your passion extends beyond the forces, that's acceptable as well as long as it's a driving force for you to effectively secure your purpose to make a change.

Before defining your lifestyle to be labeled by society, conduct your own research and decide what works for you. What matters the most is your own thoughts and desires as opposed to what society tries to force on you. Avoid judging others once you've reached a level of mastery. Consuming animal products is not just a choice but a bad habit, addiction, learned lifestyle, and occupation in some cases. Offer a solution as opposed to creating a new problem or making an existing problem worse.

Although there are rules and restraints with dietary changes, health should always be your number one priority regardless of which journey you choose. Keep that in mind when making a decision to transition. The animal rights movement is something that's very important for many reasons; however, jumping into a vegan diet blindfolded could cause you to solely rely on ultra-processed foods for nutrients. Take your time; don't rush the process. Allow your body to adjust and adapt to its new environment.

For more detailed information on the history of veganism, please visit http://vegansociety.today/. I found their site to be very helpful in locating early newsletters along with a complete historical timeline.

Part Two

What It Means To Live A Healthy Lifestyle

Chapter 4

Living a Holistic Lifestyle

"Do not let the behavior of others destroy your inner peace."
~ Dalai Lama

I remember stepping into a random holistic doctor's office desperately seeking help for the pain I could no longer bear. I was in tears begging for an answer with certainty that offered me the chance to feel better. That day was the start of a journey that would never end. Although I had some knowledge regarding the holistic approach, it was nothing compared to the knowledge I've gained over the years. I knew herbs would play a role in healing my body, but it was much more than a few herb-filled capsules, herbal tea, and a clean diet to get me back to health. I realized I had to focus on areas of my life I refused to face because they brought so much pain. I kept those thoughts locked up, but my emotions were still responding to the pain I endured that never faded. Before I could realize what was happening, I found myself in a place full of anxiety, anger, confusion, and hopelessness. Reflecting on those moments for the purpose of writing this book allowed me to see how changing my daily habits and mindset saved me from a treacherous ride to the grave.

What Is a Holistic Lifestyle?

Living a holistic lifestyle involves surrendering negative thoughts, emotions, and bad habits in order to vibrate more abundantly. A holistic lifestyle brings forth the change that manifests our purpose in this world. The limitless ability we have to improve the troubled areas in our lives makes everything about discovering the true meaning of human health phenomenal.

You can create healthy new habits to improve any area in your life that disrupts your inner peace or prevents you from being your highest self. The most common practices are yoga, meditation, self-affirmation, clean eating, exercise, and body-based methods such as massages. If you find a more effective holistic approach such as reading, writing, or speaking with a life coach, then by all means create your own healthy habits. Finding an overall balance in life is more rewarding than any seemingly peaceful disguise used to convince others.

Living Holistically

I was always in disguise trying to create a picture-perfect life. I wasn't interested in living holistically because I thought it was about health. I figured most people were interested in the lifestyle because they were sick or faced with an unexpected diagnosis. As unfortunate as I find it today, that's how I became interested. As many of us do, we confuse holistic healing (physical healing) with holistic living (emotional, spiritual, etc.). Prior to the physical challenges I've faced, I was content with wallowing in my own pity and using bad habits to cope. I had no idea I would be conducting a self-evaluation from a simple thoughtless visit to a holistic doctor seeking enough strength to get my old life back.

I can't believe my goal was to get my old life back, the life filled with emotional pain and unproductiveness. The holistic influencers I surrounded myself with encouraged me to dig deeper than the surface of things to discover what really was causing so much physical stress on my body. It was tough facing problems I covered up internally, but just like a caterpillar, I was able to come out of my cocoon as a new and improved version of myself as a gossamer-winged butterfly.

It doesn't matter how severe or complex the problem is, there'll always be a holistic approach that can help you find balance while healing from within. The only requirement is to have an open mind. You have to be receptive in allowing your truths to resurface so you can heal properly. The reason why focusing on yourself as a whole is so important is because how you feel on the inside (heart and mind) affects your overall health (physically and mentally).

How Fibromyalgia Changed My Life

I remember when I was at the peak of happiness. It was at a time when I felt like everything was happening according to God's plan and opportunities for advancement in my career were presenting themselves more frequently. I even cleaned up my credit to the point of damn near perfection and was able to purchase my first brand new car without a cosigner. I just knew the frivolous problems I had experienced in the past were the end of troubled times. Unfortunately, I couldn't have been more wrong. I started 2014 with great accomplishments and a partially fulfilled 5-year career plan. I was so hyped about how things were going that I decided to start my fitness journey after being inspired by Lauren Smith, a fitness influencer. She is such a great person to work with and I love her naturalness. I still to this day join her fitness challenges and attend local fitness events because of her authentic personality and sincerity. Although I love fitness and the health benefits of it, life taught me that if you're not careful, your pain can override your passion.

My fitness journey was short-lived due to a life-changing event. In retrospect, I wish I'd fought for what I knew was my purpose. I became pregnant and was immediately thrown off balance by everything that came with it. I was an emotional wreck, stressed, and just completely unhappy with myself. Let's just say it wasn't a pleasant experience. I spent the next three and a half years mentally, spiritually, and emotionally drained. Instead of acknowledging what was happening and doing something about it, I perceived it as typical life problems. Before I knew it, I was experiencing some serious physical changes. It started with a headache and neck pain, and by the next morning, I could barely think straight because my whole entire body ached. After two weeks of pain that wasn't subsiding, I began to reflect on the days prior. The pain started December 26, 2016. I could never forget the date because it was the day after Christmas. I remember the holidays (Thanksgiving and Christmas) being refreshing and full of exciting moments. I couldn't understand what would cause so much pain. From December 26, 2016, until mid-April 2017, I felt like the living dead. I couldn't work, couldn't care for my daughter, but most of all I couldn't find an answer to my problems (and neither could the doctor). My doctor ran a complete blood count (CBC) test and couldn't find anything. Every test they ran came back normal, which was a relief and disappointment at the same time. After being referred to a rheumatologist and having several more tests ran, they diagnosed me with Fibromyalgia. I was relieved because I thought I could take a pill and it would all go away. Sadly, I was completely wrong. All they did was treat the symptoms and follow up with me on how my body was responding to the medication.

To be candid about how I felt, I was ready to die. I was done with the doctors (yes, multiple doctors) and done with life. None of my doctors would give me confirmation that the pain would go away so I could live a normal life again. I couldn't work (which made money tight), and during the entire process I felt tortured to have to watch my daughter jump from house to house in another state because I couldn't care for her. Yes, I was ready to end it all and be thankful that I had the opportunity to actually have *good days* in my life. At that time, I resented everyone, even God. I felt like I did everything right and handled every past situation accordingly. As I begin to reflect more on the chain of events, I'm amazed at the irony of the situation. We tend to handle problems individually (treating the symptoms) instead of tackling the underlying problem(s). When I decided to look at myself as a whole and focus in on my emotional, spiritual, and mental state, I knew fibromyalgia was nothing more than a symptom of an unbalanced life. When I began to face my feelings by acknowledging how I really felt prior to the pain, how long I felt that way, and how I dealt with it, I knew my problem was deeper than I had initially thought. Once I identified those three things, I stopped handling problems "accordingly" and began to heal properly. I started to practice meditation and self-affirmations, which eventually led to yoga and, finally, back to fitness.

I slowly began to feel the pain subside. Although it took months (close to a year) for it to go away completely, it was more than what the medication was doing. It wasn't just my life problems I had to face but my diet as well. I was eating a lot of mucus-forming foods and not recognizing how my body was responding. My journey to veganism was tough love I was giving myself. As much as I would like to say all of this happened overnight, it didn't. It happened over a 5-year span that included my initial fitness journey, pregnancy, depression, fibromyalgia, and self-awareness. Once I defeated what I'd like to call the most necessary challenge in my life, I became more aware of my emotions and how I would respond to things that affected me. I also was able to discover my purpose because of the pain I experienced. When I realized health and fitness was my purpose area in life, everything became so clear and I was shocked how life showed me that. I reminisced about the days that my life was balanced and how fitness meant the world to me. I was able to see how everything (my identity and passion) just vanished because I was no longer living a balanced life. It wasn't until I found balance again that my identity and passion resurfaced.

The Late Great Dr. Sebi

I was able to turn my life around by just believing it was possible. Having faith in possibilities can be difficult when living in troubled times, and faith is even more difficult when people in your inner circle have more doubts about your plans than you. Alfredo Bowman's words of wisdom helped reduce my anxiety and gave me hope to put forth the effort to make a change. If you're unfamiliar with Alfredo Bowman (also known as Dr. Sebi) – and his practices, he's a self-educated man from the Honduran village of Ilanga. He was born on November 26, 1933, and unfortunately left us on August 6, 2016. Although he's no longer with us, his legacy lives on.

Growing up in Honduras with his family, Dr. Sebi took on unhealthy eating habits as many of us do as children. As he began to age and left Honduras to come to the United States, he found himself in a situation many people of older age do. He was diagnosed with diabetes, obesity, asthma, and ED (Erectile Dysfunction). Most men would attest that an erectile dysfunction diagnosis could be a hard pill to swallow, especially when people in your age group are still sexually active. To endure this level of emotional and physical pain all at once could lead anyone to seek help and challenge what we're often told to be impossible. Because of his eagerness to reverse his conditions, Sebi connected with a Chinese herbalist who opened his eyes to a new world of healing. After receiving the help and knowledge to reverse his existing conditions, he realized that reversing a disease is possible. It also sparked a firing desire within him to dedicate the remainder of his life to save the lives of many desperate hopeless people seeking a miracle.

I would like to point out a few vital points about Dr. Sebi's methods and beliefs.

1.) His primary focus was human health by the use of electric/ alkaline foods
2.) He was not a supporter of veganism or its recommended food groups for healthy living
3.) He did not believe in individualizing diseases. He believed in one disease which was mucus
4.) He believed in the power of herbs and its ability to alkalize the body to cure all diseases

As a follower of Dr. Sebi for many years and his approach to diseases, I found that he is most famous for reversing illnesses by his one disease approach. Most new followers are filled with curiosity on how he came to that conclusion considering the unique symptoms that are associated with every disease. I pondered it for a while too, wondering how mucus could be linked to any illnesses that are not directly affected by the over-production of mucus in the nasal mucosa, which would be obvious with a cold, flu, or sinus infection. I mean, who would argue that mucus isn't linked to a cold, flu, or even pneumonia. I was pretty concerned about his thought process in the beginning as it related to diseases, but I knew he had to be onto something considering the many lives he saved along the way. It wasn't until I binge watched his YouTube videos and studied his work that it began to make sense. He was always so quick to correct someone with his famous rebuttal

"There's only one disease and that's mucus." I received clarity when I ran across a video with him speaking with an older lady regarding a family member that was diagnosed with Alzheimer's. His response made me realize that I knew nothing more than what I could see with the naked eye, which was not much at all.

> "Alzheimer's is a brain problem. Remember, there's only one disease. When you have mucus in the nasal passage it's sinusitis; when you have mucus in the bronchial tubes it's bronchitis; when you have mucus in the lungs it's pneumonia – for you to have Alzheimer's, where's the mucus? Yes, the brain. So we have to remove the mucus from the body, especially the brain, but then we have to feed the brain. That's where biochemistry comes into play."
>
> ~ Dr. Sebi

When I began to listen to him break down how the body works, I knew that I had been completely brainwashed over the years. As a child, or even as an adult, we aren't educated by the leaders in our lives (parents, teachers, doctors, etc.) on the power of the body and how it's able to heal itself under the right conditions. We're only told what medications to take to cure a minor infection/disease, anesthetize the pain for an "incurable" disease, or what medication to take that'll provide a longer life span (in misery most likely). We are prescribed man-made pills for the most unnecessary conditions. Instead of seeking love, support, or at the very least a therapist to help discover the underlying cause of our depression and anxiety, we'll run to the doctor who'll prescribe a bottle of Xanax because he/she could care less about what caused it in the first place.

I can't express enough how important it is to become proactive about healing yourself in every aspect of your life. You don't need to have a medical degree to create a totally different trajectory for your life. I am a living witness that you'll see more results by working on yourself than giving doctors the luxury of having that much control over your life. Although I stand by this 100%, I am not suggesting that regular doctor visits aren't necessary. If you are symptomatic, please visit your primary care doctor for a diagnosis. The healthcare system we have today is effective in many ways, especially for identifying the origin of the problem. Because of this system, we're able to effectively choose a holistic approach that caters to our unique condition. Also, western medicine is sometimes necessary in extreme life or death cases. I am not suggesting that you refrain from seeking medical attention. My recommendations as it pertains to self-care are specifically for people who sought medical attention, were diagnosed, and are now seeking a holistic lifestyle that includes eastern medicine as opposed to relying on pharmaceutical medication for a lifetime.

How Dr. Robert Morse Became My Living Hope

Dr. Sebi gave me hope in knowing I had the power to heal myself, but it was Dr. Robert Morse N.D., D.Sc. M.H., who made it more of a reality for me. By the time I learned about Dr. Sebi, he had already passed away that month prior. Although I was able to research his practices and even purchase a few of his recommended herbs, I wanted more. I knew if he were still alive he would still be fighting to make a difference by teaching us to rely on the power we have within. One day, I stumbled upon one of Dr. Robert Morse's YouTube videos on fibromyalgia. I didn't have any expectations of him delivering a message I would care to listen to because I was only interested in Dr. Sebi's practices. Since I was at a point of desperation in my journey to health, I watched the video anyway. I could not believe how similar his approach was to Dr. Sebi's practices. I immediately felt fulfilled from the emptiness I felt having to rely on Dr. Sebi's videos as my motivation to continue on my journey. Dr. Morse reminded me so much of Dr. Sebi in reference to their can-do attitude in response to reversing "incurable" diseases. If you don't know Dr. Morse, he is a naturopathic doctor that believes in healing the body through detoxification. His practices are similar to Dr. Sebi's in the belief that the body is designed to heal itself under the right conditions, including what they refer to as God's herbs.

Dr. Morse recommends God's herbs as a source for detoxing the lymphatic system. Rather than focusing on one disease as Dr. Sebi did, Morse focuses on the lymphatic system and how every disease is connected to it. Detoxifying the lymphatic system is the key to getting the body to function properly. A dysfunctional circulatory system is what prevents the body from eliminating waste. The lymphatic system is an important part of the immune system and protects us from bacteria, viruses, and fungus. This is the system that fights all inflammation. For every disease or illness, the lymphatic system is somewhere involved. Dr. Morse teaches how the immune system is designed to destroy the cells that are damaged or weakened by acids through the lymph nodes. To help you understand better, The Great Lymphatic system (sewer system) is a part of the vascular system. Interstitial fluid is what surrounds the body's cells. When interstitial fluid enters the lymph capillary, it becomes lymph. Lymph carries waste and damaged cells to the lymph vessels. The lymph vessels are considered to be the sewer pipes in the body that carry waste to the appropriate chambers where they are sorted accordingly. The chambers, referred to as the septic tanks, receive the waste. Eating a highly processed diet overwhelms this system, causing the body to become extremely acidic and preventing the lymphatic system from eliminating waste. Unfortunately, medical doctors are advising that when interstitial fluid enters the lymph capillary, 10% becomes lymph and the other 90% is returned to the bloodstream. This is misleading/false because cells are not broken down in the blood.

> "The body has to get rid of cells that are damaged. When you have a stagnant dehydrated lipid based flood, that's where most of the symptoms man deals with lies. When you see this then you realize that cells must be taken and constantly broken down by macrophages in the lymph nodes, not through the blood, but through the lymph system and in the lymph nodes."
>
> ~ Dr. Robert Morse

Proceeding to elaborate on how we are misled by our healthcare system, Morse discusses in detail where waste is sent and how the body eliminates it.

> "From the lymph nodes, where does waste go? Not back into the blood system. You can convert some of this chemistry but most of it has to be eliminated to the outside world. Where do you think your body does that, through the liver? The liver doesn't expel to the outside world, but your three kidneys do. You have three kidneys that are the main eliminating organs of cellular waste, not your stool. I know some of you are thinking 'wait, three kidneys?' Yes, three Kidneys! Your skin is your largest kidney. This is simple stuff the medical doctors should be taught and should know."
>
> ~ Dr. Robert Morse

When the lymphatic system is overwhelmed by acidosis (a buildup of toxins) mainly caused by bad dietary choices, often leads to a series of bodily symptoms. Morse's approach is to eliminate waste by cleaning the lymph nodes through clean eating (fruitarian diet) and herbal medicine, not by removing lymph nodes or adding more to the buildup. Your lymphatic system is the immune system that keeps the body clean. The main focus of his protocol is to detox the body back to a state of homeostasis (a stable equilibrium).

Although Dr. Morse is known for his detox methods, he also spoke a great deal about mental health. I remember watching one of his videos where he spoke about the power of a conscious mind. A conscious mind is having a level of awareness in regards to what is happening around you and in the world. It contributes towards your perception of things and your ability to allow yourself to be receptive to physical and spiritual change. Although most naturopathic doctors focus on nutrition and herbal medicine to reverse diseases, they also believe in higher consciousness through knowledge, truth, and courage. It's just unfortunate that most people don't actually seek help until the problem becomes physical. People usually carry on with life being mentally unbalanced with no real understanding about how emotions release hormones such as cortisol, epinephrine, glucagon, etc. that directly affect our overall health.

I'm certain at this point in the book you're probably wondering "What does this have to do with veganism?" I'd be glad to explain. Most people transitioning to veganism have aspirations far beyond animal rights. They desire much more, including being at peace with the universe as well as finding mental, emotional, and sometimes financial balance. With these aspirations, a diet alone will not achieve your goals. For example, Russell Simmons discussed his transitioning journey in his book *The Happy Vegan*. I can't recall him once discussing his reasons for transitioning without mentioning his focus on finding an overall balance that benefited him entirely. He discussed yoga and meditation and how balance in different areas of his life worked together to make him a better person. He also mentioned how it allowed him to reap the benefits of a complete transformation that created a space in his life full of peace, clarity, and awareness.

Most people who are not vegan have this belief that you automatically reach an all-time high in life just by transitioning to a vegan diet. This is false in so many ways. I exercise five to six days per week, but when people see me the first thing they say is, "Oh that vegan diet is paying off!" Or, "I need to become vegan so I can look like you." They completely disregard my hard work in the gym. I've met several people in the gym who are meat eaters and have amazing physiques and they get credit for their hard work. On the other hand, I have to explain that it wasn't veganism that allowed me to see results, but my hard work in the gym and clean eating/portion control in the kitchen.

The purpose of part 2 is to enlighten you about what has to happen to achieve your physical, mental, emotional, and spiritual goals. Don't rely solely on veganism to fix your brokenness. When I made the decision to give up all animal products, I was under the impression that I would see significant changes. I just knew I would be happier, slimmer, smarter, and fit; all which turned out to be so far from the truth. Although I was a little annoyed about the reality of it, I did have an *Aha!* moment. I came to the realization that none of what I thought made any sense. How could it be possible for me improve my deficiencies without some form of practice or dedication that focuses on my trouble areas. Like a lot of us, I viewed veganism as the magic pill, but the truth is that veganism and holistic living are two totally different ways of living. In fact, there are only a few vegan diets that actually contribute toward the physical realm of a holistic lifestyle. Call me the honest vegan if you'd like, but I refuse to advise or insinuate that veganism is the key to healing anything other than physical healing and that only applies when it's a healthy vegan diet.

Living Your Best Life

We create our own reality. It's our biggest advantage in life. Your reality does not have to be what people around you want it to be. The last thing I would encourage is for you to follow a set of rules made by family, friends, or a particular community of people. Decide what changes are suitable for you that meet your expectations, and then determine what daily habits will allow you to make that your reality. I'm certain you don't want to end up in the doldrums because you presumed veganism was the key to fixing all your problems. Take time to focus on what you envision and then create daily habits to reach your level of wholeness. Be mindful there are many vegans in this world that are depressed, suicidal, unhealthy, and unfit. Although they may have adopted a vegan lifestyle, they are not eating food that nourishes the body nor are they taking the necessary steps to find the balance that leads to this purposeful happy feeling everyone speaks of. Veganism is just a title and should not set limitations on how far you soar on your journey to become the person you have always wanted to be.

If you feel that you have found balance in your life and everything is compromised by your diet, be my guest and use veganism as the final piece to your puzzle. I believe it is best that you identify why your diet is such a problem for you, define how you'd like to fix it, and explore what lifestyles align with your dietary demands. This isn't advice to force you into veganism or deter you from it, but to simply encourage you to avoid hopping from one *woke* community of people to the next. Excuse my Black English vernacular for the term *woke*, but it's a common colloquialism that means being aware and informed of what's happening around you and in the world. Everyone who claims to have knowledge on a particular issue or topic is not always speaking on the issue with the necessary level of expertise. They don't bring forth change along the magnitude that grips the core of the issue to see worthwhile results on an optimal level. Don't be a victim in a *stay woke* movement to make dietary changes just to repeat history by creating new bad eating habits along with yesterday's attitude.

Chapter 5

Nutrient Dense Foods

"When you start eating food without labels,
you no longer need to count calories."
~ Amanda Kraft

I am not a healthcare professional nor am I a nutritionist. I do not have a medical degree hanging on my wall. I have a degree in Accounting and a strong passion for fitness. Despite the career journey I embarked on, I've spent years educating myself on nutrition and the confusion surrounding healthy dieting. One misleading piece of information that adds to the confusion is the need to consume animal products to sustain a healthy diet. The progressive decline in human health over the years reveals the truth that half of the foods we consume were never meant for human consumption. Dead food does not belong in the human body. One red flag is the multitude of people in this world suffering from gastrointestinal problems. Our choices are our lifeline and when we make bad food choices we create adverse outcomes. Eating meat and dairy is another form of life support. We must eat to survive, but eating living food is what keeps us alive and well. A life of physical propensity combats our daily exposure to toxic chemicals. Allowing recommendations from people and companies to deter us from living an unorthodox lifestyle is an action that keeps us all trapped in this toxic norm. Even today's USDA food reco-mmendations and dietary guidelines, promote a system that's designed to keep us trapped, allowing companies in the meat and dairy industry to use our eating addictions to make money.

Deprogramming takes time to reverse the mind control our system has on us. It's designed to channel all its energy in creating addictions that are hard to break. Promoting a diet for nutritional needs and hunger is now a disguise to eat for pleasure. Being a cautious eater sounds easy, but the dependency on food for satisfaction is the new trigger to eat when experiencing high emotions. From an aggressive physiological spectrum, some people use food as an antidepressant when battling depression, anxiety, or a bipolar disorder. Sadly, high emotions are just one part of it all; people associate food with every aspect of their lives. Birthdays are associated with cake and ice cream, Thanksgiving with turkey, stuffing, and dressing; 4th of July with cookouts (hotdogs, hamburgers, fish fry, etc.); and Valentine's Day with chocolate. Those are bad habits and addictions we've created in the human diet.

A new standard for future generations regarding health and wellness is the most powerful move to make. Today's emphasis on health and wellness is obstructed by gimmicks and get rich schemes. Take veganism, for example. Companies are now capitalizing on the vegan movement by selling ultra-processed foods to promote the idea of a healthier alternative. It's disturbing for a number of reasons. The number one reason is the confusion it creates in individuals who feel empowered to make changes based on false presumptions. It becomes too complex for them to grasp because they have this preconceived notion of what health is and how to obtain it. When they realize how processed foods don't help them, their presumptions are shattered due to a lack of results. This could annihilate their hopes of one day obtaining optimal health.

I will never forget sitting with a friend on a curb near a chop shop in Orangeburg, South Carolina after attending a college party. We were so drained that we sat on the curb and waited until we built up our energy to walk to the car. We sat and talked about everything from career goals to personal goals. While sharing her aspirations, she reached in her purse and grabbed a protein bar that looked familiar to me. It was familiar because I would often read the nutrition label for the different flavors for that brand as something to do while waiting in line to purchase gas at the gas station. She ripped the wrapper off, took a bite, and looked at me and said, "I've been good about keeping healthy food in my purse." I knew she was trying to make better choices, so I encouraged her to stay motivated. I knew that protein bar was full of fats, sugar, and simple carbs. She had faith that those bars would help her, but in actuality it was causing more harm than good. It's a tragedy being conditioned to believe that our body is made to endure the damage caused by inflammatory foods. We're resilient beings, but not that resilient.

Believe it or not, if it's sold in our grocery stores and restaurants, people will eat it without thought. This conditioned mindset from so many people in this world reflects a lack of knowledge and understanding. Some people have no clue what nutrient dense foods are. As long as we continue to eat for pleasure as opposed to nourishment and fuel, we'll forever be in this unhealthy cycle. I personally know the disadvantages because I've been that person who associated food with celebration as well as emotional quick fixes. I know how hard it is to shake those bad habits, but I also studied and now know how purposeful eating has lifelong benefits and will always beat those short pleasurable moments.

What Are Nutrient-Dense Foods?

It's typical to seek change after something bad happens. We never seek change until we are forced to deal with the consequences of our bad habits. These consequences might make the journey a little more challenging, but it won't be impossible. The fact that you are reading this book shows you are taking the initiative to educate yourself to make a change for the better. With that being said, let's jump into it.

In the beginning of this chapter, I mentioned the effects of eating dead food. Because I'm vegan, it may seem as if I'm referring to actual dead food such as meat. Although meat does apply, I'm referring to foods that have little nutritional value in the human diet. To keep the body functioning properly, you need to consume nutrient-rich foods that are primarily low in calories and high in nutrients. These foods are easy to identify and are often found in the frozen fruits and vegetables aisle, produce aisle, and random aisles that hold grains, dry beans, oils, nuts, and seeds. To prevent possible confusion when conducting your own research, there are nutrient-dense foods that are also calorie dense. Please ensure you eat those foods in moderation or smaller portions.

Reading a plethora of information on a balanced diet can lead to discouragement. The meaning of a balanced diet varies from person to person since we all have specific needs. It's just a matter of providing you with a wide range of information for you to decipher what works for you based on your specific needs. An ideal start would be to track how many calories you eat per day, then measuring how many calories you should consume per day by calculating your BMR (basal metabolic rate). You can use this information to create your meal plan to ensure that you stay within your normal caloric range. This is not required but helpful in understanding your daily macronutrients (protein, carbs, and fats) while observing how your body responds to it. You'll then be able to make adjustments if necessary until you're comfortable enough to eat intuitively.

The benefits of knowing your calorie intake is discovering your normal range. Every person is unique. My body type may require more daily calories than your body type. Depending on your fitness goals, you will find it easier to put yourself in a caloric surplus or a caloric deficit. When weight gain or health challenges present themselves, you are able to see clearly what adjustments need to be made to cater to your condition. You will be forced to choose your foods wisely and consume more fulfilling foods that are low in calories. Since overeating is prevalent, tracking your macronutrients can ease the challenge of figuring out what foods should and shouldn't be included in your meal plan. Everything that's healthy can't be included in your daily meals, so compromising one thing for another is a component of being a cautious eater. An area where most problems derive with dieting is incorporating calorie-dense foods. Avocado, legumes, oils, and nuts are calorie-dense foods that should be substituted or consumed in smaller portions. It's difficult to practice portion control with calorie-dense foods because they are not fulfilling in smaller portions.

If you're unsure how to measure nutrient density, start reading the label on the items you purchase and factor them in when preparing your meals. If one particular item such as oils or nuts takes away a large portion of your daily fats, then that's an indicator to substitute it for something else. If the label has a long list of ingredients, including things that are unfamiliar to you, then that's another indicator to explore other options. Generally, the majority of the grocery items you purchase should consist of 1-3 ingredients.

Vitamins and Minerals

We mistake a lot of things as common knowledge, but common sense is not always common. Most people are familiar with vitamin A, B, C, D, E, etc., but few people are informed about what their contributing health factors are. To tell someone to incorporate more of a particular vitamin in their diet is not helping them at all. It doesn't require much knowledge to go to Wal-Mart or a local farmer's market to look for a bottle labeled vitamin B or multivitamin to supplement. Sometimes supplementing is the best option when you're deficient and need that jump start, but supplements can prevent you from discovering what foods naturally provide what you need. When I discovered I was severely vitamin D deficient, of course I supplemented, but I was curious as well. I wanted to know everything there was to know about vitamin D and how I could naturally consume it without relying on supplements. I was surprised to learn that vitamin D is a hormone and could have contributed to the severe body aches I was experiencing. These are things I wouldn't know if I hadn't taken the time to do my research. Discovering little details like this made it less difficult for me to eat healthier. It took a few unpleasant experiences for me to get my act together and take my diet and exposure to sunlight more seriously. I catered to my body for months, treating it as if it were a newborn baby. Along my path to self-love and self-education, I became astonished yet frightened at my past ability to take my mental health and physical health for granted for so long.

The old famous quote "knowledge is power" has a whole new meaning to me. I get chills comparing my old uneducated ways of thinking to my new knowledgeable, free-spirited mindset. Extraordinary things happen every day, but nothing compared to the things that manifest from a mind full of wisdom.

Being intrigued by everything I discovered, I was hungry for more. I wasn't as well versed on minerals as I wanted to be, so I did the research and used my leisure time to soak up all the information. Dr. Sebi's words of wisdom were the muse that aroused my curiosity. He enlightened me how to consume minerals in abundance by adding sea moss to my diet. I was so in tune with everything I was learning that my kitchen became my place of peace filled with herbs and spices. I wanted to experience the benefits of that part of nature that we all take for granted. My desires to become one with nature led to my fascination with herbs. The great thing about herbs is that they're packed with minerals and are easy to consume in different forms (tea, smoothie, capsules, etc.). Could you imagine drinking a cup of herbal tea or a sea moss smoothie consuming more than 90 minerals in one sitting? That's more than what most people consume per day.

Minerals are broken down into two types: trace minerals and macro minerals. Each type is equally important but differs in quantity. The term trace, as you may know, means a small quantity so only a small amount of these minerals is needed daily (less than 1mg per day). Copper, Zinc, Manganese, Iodine, Chromium, Sulfur, and Selenium are a few trace minerals.

Macro minerals require a larger quantity per day. Many people are familiar with macro-minerals since they are mentioned more often. Potassium, Calcium, Magnesium, Sodium, Chloride, etc. are all macro minerals. Most whole foods contain these minerals and are easily accessible.

Superfoods

You may have heard the term superfoods one time or another throughout life, but what are superfoods? They are foods packed with nutrients that provide a wide range of health benefits. They are not limited to a particular food group and provide desirable results when consumed daily. Juicing has helped me with consuming superfoods in bulk. Of course, organic foods are the most beneficial; however, if you can't afford organic foods don't beat yourself up. You can still reap the benefits. Superfoods include:

- ➤ Avocado
- ➤ Berries (strawberries, blackberries, blueberries, etc.)
- ➤ Almonds
- ➤ Kale
- ➤ Ginger
- ➤ Turmeric
- ➤ Flaxseeds
- ➤ Sweet Potatoes

There are other superfoods that are non-vegan which, in my opinion, are not reliable sources. An example would be raw milk. I'm unsure why we promote raw milk as a reliable superfood source considering the bad bacteria it carries, along with the risk of major health challenges. While learning the benefits of healthy foods, do not get caught up on the label. Some superfoods should be consumed in moderation due to the sugar content and other added ingredients. The term superfood is just used to describe nutrient-rich foods that are packed with vitamins and minerals. If you're on a whole foods diet and eat pretty clean already, searching for healthier alternatives is unnecessary.

Antioxidants

What are antioxidants? Let's first discuss what oxidants are and why we've become so anti- towards them. Oxidants are molecules that are highly reactive in their role of damaging other molecules. They are often referred to as free radicals, but oxidants and free radicals are not the same. They are used interchangeably because they both steal electrons; however, their abilities are much different. Free radicals are unstable molecules that are missing elections or a single electron. They become highly reactive in stealing electrons from other healthy cells causing them to become weakened and damaged. Considering this chain reaction, yes, free radicals act as oxidants because they steal electrons from other cells; however, they are also able to do the opposite by giving up electrons. They are able to act as a reducing agency which is opposite from oxidants. Although oxidants and free radicals are used for healthy immune function, oxidative stress can lead to serious health challenges due to the increase of damaged cells and the body's inability to counteract it. This is usually in result of things like smoking, ultra-processed foods, inflammation, alcohol, etc. Antioxidants are naturally present in the body; however, they can be overpowered by free radicals, leading to an increase of inflammation in the body.

Luckily, we are able to prevent and reduce the adverse effects of oxidative stress by becoming cautious eaters and choosing a healthier lifestyle. These choices will allow our body to neutralize free radicals while increasing our chance of preventing or reversing an existing disease. Antioxidants act as a reducing agents/stabilizers in the body by donating electrons, which ultimately ends the chain reaction. A plant-only diet consists of foods high in antioxidants and would probably be the best source to increase your intake. To avoid oxidative stress, creating an environment that allows the body to fight against harmful invaders that damage healthy cells is a small action that makes a huge difference.

Caloric Surplus v. Caloric Deficit

Calorie density is the most overlooked part of the equation that represents 100% of how the body responds. It's also the key to creating a caloric deficit or a caloric surplus. This could require you to go through different stages of relatively low calories to fairly high calories, all of which are techniques to train the body to respond in a way that aligns with your goals. Measuring calorie density is critical because it applies to your diet as a whole and does not exempt healthy foods that are calorie dense. Most people fail miserably at dieting because the foods they consume are unfulfilling calorie dense foods. Nutrient density has gained so much attention that it's often forgotten that the weight of our food is just as important in reference to a realistic lifestyle change. Eating for volume should always be the goal when decreasing calories otherwise you can expect periodic moments of binge eating which will start the cycle of yo-yo dieting.

There are certain healthy foods I recommend you avoid when cutting calories due to the decrease in volume and the absence of satiety. Satiety is the feeling of fullness after eating a meal that eliminates the feeling of hunger for a period of time. To provide more clarity, raw nuts (walnuts, almonds, etc.) and zucchini provide vital nutrients, but the difference between the two is volume. Raw walnuts are 2,966 calories per pound, meaning you would have to decrease your portion size just to stay in a caloric deficit. Zucchini, on the other hand, is 76 calories per pound, so increasing your portion size isn't a problem while remaining in a caloric deficit. Other healthy calorie-dense fats are olive oil (3,998 calories per pound) and tahini (2,691 calories per pound). Using nuts from the example I gave, the calories could be much higher if they are covered in chocolate, caramel, or powdered sugar, making it more difficult to sustain a caloric deficit. When peanuts are processed to nut butters and almonds are processed to almond flour, the likelihood of overeating is at its highest. One to two tablespoons of healthy nutrient-dense fats can take you out of a caloric deficit into a caloric surplus easily.

Eating in a caloric surplus does not only result in weight gain, but also creates conditions internally that causes the body to generate inflammation. An increased appetite is rarely to blame for binge eating or eating in a caloric surplus. I had my share of challenges believing that was the case, but I realized although I was eating healthy foods, I wasn't eating for volume. I was merely eating smaller portions of the foods I enjoyed which was not fulfilling at all. At first I would binge eat once every two weeks, but then it began to happen more frequently. When I started to increase the amount of calorie-dense foods in my diet, the more severe my hunger was. My urge to binge eat would last a few days initially, but sadly those few days turned into weeks, months, and then years of struggling with portion control. My tunnel vision to focus on healthy foods kept me from reaching a healthy medium.

For unrelated reasons, I increased my water consumption because that's what everyone said I should do. All I heard during my fitness journey was "Stay hydrated! Stay hydrated!" so that's what I did. When I made that change it all came together full speed. My appetite noticeably decreased and satiety signals shifted drastically. The girl who once struggled with portion control had to set her alarm to ensure she didn't miss a meal. That was an exciting moment for me and drinking a minimum of 1 gallon per day became a matter of principle.

My mom's matter of principle was the opposite. When I was a kid my mom had a rule: eat before you drink. In retrospect, it makes perfect sense considering my recent enlightenment, but then I couldn't grasp it. I felt as if it was a punishment to force me and my siblings to obey her at all times. How foolish of me to be blinded by her true motive. It wasn't to punish us in any way, but to ensure we ate the majority of the food on our plate before filling ourselves up with water and losing our appetite. Her motive was about saving money and not allowing us to waste food. Reflecting on this made me realize that we're not always hungry but dehydrated. The most fulfilling foods such as zucchini, celery, lettuce, and cucumber have high water content consisting of more than 70% water. Making little adjustments with food choices and shopping for a realistic lifestyle change makes all the difference. My advice to those who share similar challenges is to incorporate or increase hydrating foods in your diet for volume to control your urges. You'll be amazed at the results.

Now that you know what to do, the next step is training your body for it. The uncut truth about increasing your water intake is the challenge of actually doing it and being consistent. Of course, drinking a glass of water is easy, but drinking a gallon every day is where the challenge resides. When I started to increase my water intake, I found it extremely difficult because my body wasn't used to it. After spending years filling myself up with Mountain Dew, Sprite, sweet tea, and orange soda, my taste buds were rejecting every drop of water I would drink. I was only able to drink a half of gallon per day until my taste buds adjusted to the change. Let's just say I was on the deep end of an unhealthy journey. Once my body became acclimated to the change, I never looked back. I would load up on water throughout the day because I knew how far I've come to improve my health. Eating for volume was the final piece to my puzzle.

Keeping this pertinent information in mind, there are still other factors to consider. When eating in a caloric deficit, avoid cutting your calories below 1,200. Cutting calories that low will not expedite your fitness journey, but could lead to an unhealthy relationship with food and potential health problems. The only exception for this extreme measure is if it's carefully monitored by healthcare professionals for unique circumstances. This may not apply to those who participate in body-building competitions as some extreme measures are taken to get stage ready. Even considering this, it should be discussed with your coach to ensure you are taking proper steps to manage it.

A caloric surplus is an unfavorable lifestyle choice but is perceived differently in the fitness world. A lot of professional bodybuilders are eating in a caloric surplus during bulking season to build muscles that they can expose later during cutting season. Many revert to a clean bulk, which means retaining a clean/healthy diet while increasing portion size; hence increasing calories.

A dirty bulk, on the other hand, would be increasing your protein but also incorporating more unhealthy foods for satisfaction. Both methods work equally to help build muscle, but more body fat is gained in a dirty bulk which varies depending on your body type. The objective for most is to eventually shed the body fat. It's an ongoing cycle of transitioning from a caloric surplus to a caloric deficit. It may seem like an interesting process, but don't get it mistaken; although professional bodybuilders overeat intentionally, it is not always a healthy process.

If you haven't noticed yet, I've touched on every area of a healthy balanced lifestyle, and food is the common denominator. Without health, nothing can be achieved in life. Good health allows you to pursue your dreams at an unstoppable level. Good health enables you to think clearer to make wiser decisions, meet the physical demands of your career choice, save money, live in a healthier environment, and influence those around you. If you don't understand this yet, it's because you haven't experienced life on the other side. When your health fails you, it's a near death experience because your life is at a standstill. Being in a physical state that hinders you from living a purposeful life makes you reconsider your choices. I'm thankful that prior to discovering my purpose, I was able to get a taste of what it's like not being able to jump out the bed, take a shower, and get dressed to go to work and enjoy my day. It's a horrific experience that feels like you're living to die and desperately dying to live.

Processed Foods

*"Learning how to choose the right foods within
each nutrient category is one of the keys to long-term success."*
~ Maya Adams, M.D.

There are three types of food options: fresh organic foods, processed foods, and ultra-processed foods. Fresh organic foods are consumed in their natural form with no added preservatives or genetic modifications. Processed food is anything that has been changed from its natural form prior to consumption (frozen, blanched, cooked, canned, genetically modified, etc.). Processed foods are not necessarily unhealthy but because it's a term commonly used to describe unhealthy food choices, people often apply that notion to all foods that are considered processed. Ultra-processed foods, on the other hand are the center of concern. It's the cause of many health challenges. These foods contain empty calories that are high in sugar, sodium, simple carbs, and unhealthy fats. Because ultra-processed foods are calorie dense, it's difficult to practice portion control. They are labeled with a long list of ingredients with fancy packaging to make them more appealing. In reality, there's nothing healthy about these foods. Some products can be misleading with things like gluten-free, soy-free, and zero cholesterol to make you believe they are healthy. Falling for those traps can prevent you from managing your hunger and staying consistent. I wouldn't suggest eliminating labeled foods from your diet, but minimizing the amount of packaged foods you purchase at your market will help. By doing this you'll have a better grip on controlling bad eating habits.

*"If you're eating an average American diet, chances are you're eating
too many ultra-processed foods and those foods are adding more sugar
to your diet than you would expect."*
~ Robin Shreeves

Very few people desire to give up ultra-processed foods, including vegans. Since we weren't born in a world that strives to live for health and not wealth, we have little control over the unhealthy things that are tempting and readily available to us. Instead, we are evolving into a world of convenience. Companies are creating new ways to make meals quick, easy, and on the go, with little concern about how added perspectives and harmful ingredients affect human health.

Nutrition Facts

"Food is alive and should eventually die and a food that doesn't is something we should worry about. It's been over processed; it's been hyper processed."

~ Michael Pollan

If most of your foods have months or years of shelf life, that's a red flag that you're not on the right track. From one perspective, you may find it beneficial to load up at the grocery and not have to worry about food spoiling before you have a chance to cook it. I agree that it does help with saving money; however, that's what companies want you to believe: that you're saving money while eliminating the frequent trips to the market to purchase more fresh food for your family. It's convenient, and that's the aim of companies in the food industry. The trick about it is it's in exchange for your good health. You have to ask yourself if the frequent trips to the grocery store cause that much frustration and inconvenience that it's worth compromising your health. I'm at the market twice a week and although I hate it sometimes, it's part of my weekly schedule so I have gotten used to it. I know that my health is all that matters, so I'm willing to inconvenience myself for the moment rather than deal with the consequences of my bad habits.

My friends would laugh and often make fun of me because I read food labels religiously. I'm at a point where I'll read the label on products I purchase on the regular only because it's a habit I started. There are certain things I look at when purchasing certain products.

For example, if I'm at the market buying bread or noodles, the first thing I look at is the carbs. Then, I look at the ingredients to ensure it doesn't contain animal products. If I'm ok with what I see, then I begin to look at other things like sodium, fat, calories, etc. My process of what I look for in particular products is not something everyone does, nor is there a right way to do it. Some may decide to look at the calories and serving size first to decide if it's worth looking into further in regards to cholesterol, sugar, protein, etc. Everyone has different deal-breakers because some people have to consider things others don't such as nuts, milk, sodium, and fats for allergies or existing health complications. For personal reasons or fitness goals, some people may be focused on their macronutrients (fats, carbs, and protein). Whatever your process, please know that it's perfect for you as long as there is a balance of healthy fats, complex carbs, protein, and you are within normal range of your calorie and sodium intake per day.

Honestly, everything on the label is important to me. I refuse to go over 1.300mg of sodium per day, 20g of sugar per day, and 200g of carbs per day. I also ensure I stay under 1,600 calories per day to maintain my figure. These are just my numbers and should vary by person based on activity level, goals, gender, and health conditions. Below is how the Nutrition Facts appears on most packages.

Nutrition Facts

Serving Size

Amount Per Serving

Calories 0

	% Daily Values*
Total Fat 0g	0%
Saturated Fat 0g	0%
Trans Fat 0g	
Cholesterol 0mg	0%
Sodium 0mg	0%
Total Carbohydrate 0g	0%
Dietary Fiber 0g	0%
Sugars 0g	
Protein 0g	0%

The ingredients will be listed either above or below the Nutrition Facts label. If you are practicing veganism you should find ingredients such as milk and eggs in bold to ensure you avoid those products.

Along my journey to veganism I've learned a lot about reading food labels. I realized that most ingredients are listed separately because they are common food allergens. When I first became vegan, I used to believe that section was specifically for people on a vegan or keto diet. I know that sounds ridiculous for the most part, but if you never been a cautious eater then you're not privy to things like that because it doesn't apply to your lifestyle. The list of common allergenic foods are separate from the ingredients and listed under *contains*. You will find foods such as wheat, soy, milk, eggs, and nuts listed under this section.

Food Variety for a Well-Balanced Diet

When exploring new foods on a healthy diet, we tend to only eat a particular item until we're sick of it. That is not the way to go. You should eat a wide variety of foods because they all offer different vitamins and minerals that our body needs daily. Eating bananas or just blueberries all day is not a great way to start a healthy lifestyle. It's a quick way to lose interest and subconsciously set unwanted limitations. You don't want to become so disgusted with your favorite healthy foods because you made it your only option for the past 4-5 days. Due to the constant abuse to our taste buds with salty and sugary foods, it's difficult for us to enjoy healthy foods without added ingredients for taste. I know you may have heard this already but keep your plate/bowl as colorful as possible. It takes time to retrain your taste buds to adjust to your new lifestyle. With time and consistency, you'll discover that something you may not be interested in today may become your favorite food in the future. A lot of fruits and vegetables are tasty, but we have exhausted our taste buds to the point that if our meal is not packed with salt or sugar it's hard to enjoy.

It takes approximately 10-14 days to retrain your taste buds to enjoy new foods. This is not to say you won't crave your favorite unhealthy dish anymore, but you'll begin to taste your food without the extra ingredients. It's up to you to take advantage when that time arrives to continue to eat a clean diet without revisiting those bad eating habits.

I remember when I began to retrain my taste buds when I started eating a clean diet. After approximately three weeks I started treating myself again. Before I knew it, I was stuck back in my old eating habits. I realized that having a treat once in a while wasn't the best practice for me. I had to cut all snacks until I gained more control. I researched different tips and applied what I learned to permanently make a change. Sometimes I'll have a treat and don't eat it at all because my mind and taste buds just don't desire it anymore. The best method is to not feed or tease your weaknesses. Wait until you reach a point where you have more control over what you eat then treat yourself.

I've become more knowledgeable over the past four years and grateful I've managed to turn my life around before encountering permanent damage from my bad eating habits. I want this book to encourage you to become a better version of you. You can achieve whatever you put your mind to. It can be challenging initially, but your biggest challenge is telling yourself NO when temptation comes knocking at your door. This isn't just a decision you're making for your life but for your family, especially your children. Most times it's our family members who suffer the most when we're sick. Let's end the cycle of blaming it on genetics and blame it on the decisions we make every day with our food choices. Train your children to build healthy eating habits so they won't have to struggle with their health or their journey to optimal health. Proactive behavior starts today, not tomorrow, not next week, not when I finish reading this book, but right now. At this moment, make the decision to make your next meal your first meal on your new journey to health. Find an accountability partner and take charge of your future.

Chapter 6

Raw Food v. Cooked Food

"Raw food is the best way to have the cleanest energy."
~ Woody Harrelson

The conversation about raw food versus cooked food has become an ongoing discussion that grabbed my attention. It's entertaining to hear the different perspectives on the topic, but I believe the truth lies among those who experienced it. I went cold turkey on a raw vegan diet, so I know the advantages and disadvantages. Although the food withdrawals were the worst, I don't know how life would have been if I hadn't taken that step. I was suffering from severe body aches and the medication prescribed was garbage. When I decided to have an optimistic attitude about my situation, I put my mind and body in a state of receptiveness. At a point in my life with nothing to lose, I decided to take a leap of faith and try it out. Within a few months, my symptoms were nearly gone. My mobility improved and I was back to feeling well as if nothing happened. Even today if I experience a headache or minor body aches that doesn't go away within 3-4 days, I either fast or go on a raw vegan diet until it improves. Four months was the longest I've gone on a raw diet so I'm unable to attest to it being a sustainable lifestyle.

There are different approaches to a raw vegan diet, so my approach may yield different results than the typical one. When I embarked on my journey, I only included fruit, water, nuts, seeds, and herbs. It was primarily liquid based (juicing) and contained smaller amounts of nuts and seeds. I decided not to include vegetables in my diet because they are harder to digest. I'm unsure if it makes a difference, but I find it more effective for the body to heal itself that way. This isn't to say that there's no other way to see results, but to simply share my experience and how it worked for me.

There will always be a devil's advocate for every dietary lifestyle so I don't allow outside influences to deter me. The argument against a raw vegan diet is that it's not scientifically proven that raw foods are healthier than cooked foods. Since I've converted years ago I've learned not to rely on our government to tell me what works or what's true. There's still this big debate on rather the earth is round or flat, but in my opinion it'll forever be a mystery. What I admire the most about a holistic lifestyle is the freedom to rely on history, evidence, and personal experiences rather than science. Because I never practiced a raw vegan diet over a period of years, I'm unable to give a confident response on the long-term advantages or disadvantages. What I am confident in saying is eating a raw vegan diet at least once or twice per week is more effective than eating cooked food every day.

As I gain more knowledge about the body's needs and capabilities, it becomes indisputable to me that eating every day throughout the day is overkill. As ridiculous as it may sound, we could benefit from missing a day or two from eating each week. Fasting should be a major part of the human practice. It's like recharging a battery before using it the next 24 hours. My experience with fasting showed me how refreshing it is to give my body a break. Raw foods and fasting help reduce inflammation in the body which allow the body to heal itself. In many cases it's not about the food you consume and all the nutrients that food provides, but the absence of food that allows the body to boost stem cell regeneration.

Dr. Michael Greger once said, "It's not what you eat—it's what you absorb." Eating a variety of food high in nutrients is not always the answer. Detoxification can help break the barriers that create challenges with nutrition absorption. B-12 is an example I used in chapter one regarding common misconceptions. Issues people experience are not always due to the absence of B-12 in their diet, but their body's inability to absorb it. You can eat a large quantity of B-12 foods along with supplementing, but if your body is not absorbing it, you will continue to struggle with this deficiency.

Damage to your intestines or the presence of certain diseases can lead to malabsorption. B-12 is concerning for people who have doubts about the vegan diet; however, there are other concerning vitamin deficiencies that are detrimental to a person's overall health. If you want good health, focus on your gut. Everyone has their opinions about fasting and what the body needs every 3-4 hours, but the digestive system is always working to digest the food we eat. Every once in a while our digestive system needs a break. When animals get sick, most of them won't eat until the virus or bacterial infection pass. Naturally that applies to humans as well. If you haven't noticed by now, you tend to lose your appetite when you're sick. That isn't a strange thing the body does but a natural part of our healing process. It's a signal that the digestive system needs a break to preserve all its energy to heal the body. As soon as your body sends a signal to stop eating and you listen, it seems like everyone has an opinion about your decision saying things like "you need to eat something!" It could be 24 hours and everyone will swear you're starving yourself and won't be able to survive much longer.

Before you had a chance to experience the benefits, you took the bait and stuffed your face with food. Eating more will not heal your body; it will only force your digestive system to use all its energy to digest the food. Listen to your body, not to people.

Fasting

People often associate fasting with religious practices/spiritual beliefs but the benefits are equally physical as they are spiritual. Practicing regularly on a 16-hour to 24-hour fast has long-term health benefits. The obvious benefit is stabilizing insulin levels, although weight loss tends to be the primary focus for someone who is trying to detox to lose weight. The body will put up a fight but will adjust over a short period of time. During a fast, your stomach will shrink, allowing you a fresh start to practice portion control. One day of fasting does it for some people, but for others, it may take a few times of fasting to feel the difference. Below are seven health benefits from fasting:

1.) Weight Loss
2.) Cell Regeneration
3.) Regenerate Immune System
4.) Lower Sugar Levels
5.) Assist in Reversing Diseases
6.) Increase Focus
7.) Eliminate Waste

Fasting heals the mind as well as the body. I realized that I gained more confidence to achieve my career and personal goals by fasting. Not because it improves brain function, but because I was able to experience my ability to remain self-disciplined with something I found difficult to abstain from. I still have the urge to eat when fasting, but my ability to keep self-control with the presence of the urge is my natural high. It's an act of proving to myself over and over again that I can do anything I put my mind to when striving to be a better version of myself.

If you have no pre-existing health conditions and practice fasting safely, then you would think hunger would be the only feeling of discomfort. Unfortunately, that is not the case for everyone. Depending on how bad your diet was prior to fasting, you may experience withdrawals. Some people may have more symptoms than others, but that doesn't mean you are not fit to fast. If you are just starting to fast, you may experience headaches, stomach pain, nausea, and weakness. I've experienced all the above, but my body eventually adapted to my new lifestyle and now I don't have those symptoms when fasting. I do NOT suggest that you fight through the symptoms, especially if they are severe. Instead, shorten the timeframe until your body becomes comfortable. Gradually increase the number of hours until you reach your goal. Your goal could range from a 24-hour fast per week, to a 3-day or 21-day fast twice a year.

To the newbies excited to try out fasting, I will give you a disclaimer: it is difficult! I won't lie and say it's a mind thing because that's far from the truth. Your body will respond to any changes you make that affect its process to maintain homeostasis. Your thoughts have nothing to do with how the body chooses to respond. You can't think your way out of experiencing symptoms. The spiritual aspect only runs so deep. Thinking back on my journey, I can't tell you how many times I failed at fasting. It took persistence, time, and mental control to master it. You have to be mindful that your body is used to eating every day throughout the day at a certain time. If you even attempt to disrupt that process, your brain will respond, causing physical and emotional symptoms.

Drug addicts are known for going through withdrawals when attempting to quit. Most will check themselves into rehab for professional help. The other alternative exercised is gradually reducing their dosage to wean themselves off the drug to avoid severe withdrawal symptoms.

Drug use affects brain function, which affects the entire body. When used over a period of time, the body adjusts to those changes by finding a new level of balance to maintain homeostasis. Everything is affected in this process including the hormonal and nervous system. Depending on the drug and the body's high tolerance for it, the body can become dependent. The journey to recovery in this scenario is the worst because unfortunately the body is so dependent upon that drug that a person has to be exposed to it in order to function. The absence of the drug can be life threatening due to severe withdrawals such as delirium tremens. I know this is an outrageous comparison, but I wanted to explain how doing something to better yourself or improve your overall health comes with a price and that price is often challenging. The withdrawal can make you question if you're making the right decision, but that is a normal reaction!

Should I Eat Raw Herbs?

How pleasant would it be to consume herbs raw? I'm obsessed with consuming foods in their natural form but because of the human digestive inabilities, this is not the safest approach. Most herbs consist of hard seeds, wood, bark, etc. that should not be eaten raw. Even grounding the herbs could cause problems that lead to an upset stomach. Herbs are commonly sold in a few different forms: tincture, capsule, and tea. Depending on the potency, a smaller dosage is recommended to avoid any unwanted side effects.

Known for their anti-inflammatory properties, each herb has its own specific health benefits. For example, Brahmi helps improve nervous system and brain function, while dandelion caters to the improvement of organ function. There is a long list of herbs and spices that contribute to a healthy functioning body. With the right concoction of herbs, some diseases don't stand a chance of surviving in the human body. Most herbalists, including Dr. Sebi, consider it to be the key to eradicating all diseases. Although herbs are known for healing properties, they are useless without the proper diet. The food consumed is what creates the internal environment for the herbs to be effective.

Believing in Your Own Observation

I spoke on my experience on a raw vegan diet and how it helped me defeat my challenges to push through to heal physically. I had disbeliefs but I had nothing to lose and I wanted to see improvement. I got the results I wanted and experienced withdrawals as I expected. This does not have to be your story to improve your health. Your approach should be catered to your specific needs. I found that most of the information I received from holistic subject matter experts were beneficial once I actually applied it. There were some things that I tried that did not work for me and that is something I expected as well. There are a few studies that highlight how a raw vegan diet is beneficial for fibromyalgia patients, but if this disease does not apply to your medical history or current condition, then this approach may not get you the same results.[11] The point of mentioning these different holistic approaches and lifestyle changes is to educate you on healthier alternatives that heal the body and isn't used as a temporary physical fix like pharmaceutical medicine. Pharmaceutical drugs are nothing more than a form of life support for conditions medical doctors claim to be irreversible.

---

[11] Donaldson MS1, Speight N, Loomis S., *Fibromyalgia syndrome improved using a mostly raw vegetarian diet: an observational study*.PubMed.gov, (2001)

Try taking baby steps with some of these approaches to see how your body responds. A week or two is not long enough to see results, so give your body time to respond to a raw vegan diet, fasting, or herbal treatment. Whatever it is, do not let anyone else's experience change your mind. Use your own experience to determine if it's the best fit for you and your goals. Make sure you avoid consuming the same type of raw foods and herbs; focus on variety. Incorporate a wide variety of herbs, vegetables, and fruit in your diet over a period of time to better evaluate your experience.

Bodily Response and Tolerance

In a normal functioning body, our main organs, lymphatic system, immune system, and nervous system play the same role. The immune system helps fight invaders (diseases, bacteria, fungus, etc.) with the help of our lymphatic system. There is nothing surprising about that, but what is interesting is one person's tolerance for something maybe another person's intolerance. I cannot eat mango without my entire face breaking out in rashes. I really couldn't figure out why this was happening to me and not to my friends or family members. After doing some research, I discovered that mangos are from the same plant family as poison ivy. This plant family is called Anacardiaceae. I found that mangos and poison ivy share the same oily liquid substance known as urushiol which is found in the skin of mangos. Poison ivy affected me often as a kid, so it all made sense.

Mangos have caused me some very bad days, but I never felt the fruit was unhealthy. My hypersensitivity to mangos shouldn't be evidence to you that it is not meant for human consumption. Most people eat them every day and never experience an allergic reaction. Because they don't, it enables them to reap the health benefits of consuming them. This goes for many other allergens that are more common such as peanuts. Observe your own experience to dietary changes. The voice of someone else's experience should not prevent you from trying it yourself.

Fruitarians

There are a million ways to diet. None should be considered the most effective because of our environment, hypersensitivity to certain foods, and health condition. A diet that works perfectly for someone else may not benefit you. I spoke on a raw fruitarian diet briefly because it's a path I took to recovery. I didn't choose this approach based on instinct, but based on its benefits for my health condition. A fruitarian diet could consist of fruits entirely or include small portions of nuts, seeds, or veggies for nutritional purposes. Usually a fruitarian diet is practiced for a specific reason that varies by person. It is the least popular approach to dieting because of the criticism surrounding health concerns.

Healthcare professionals are somewhat against this lifestyle because they believe it is extreme and detrimental to one's health. The lack of protein, fats, and the increase in sugar content could be a dangerous lifestyle that leads to malnourishment along with high exposure to certain diseases like diabetes or dental health problems. People who choose this diet usually include nuts and seeds, but they use fruit as the main course of each meal. Contrary to popular belief, naturopathic Dr. Robert Morse has been expressing the healing capabilities in only consuming fruit. Based on studies surrounding human anatomy, Dr. Morse refers to humans as frugivores, people who primarily feed on fruits in addition to a small portion of nuts, seeds, roots, and veggies. The idea that we're designed to primarily consume fruit was from what we know about the history of early species.

Humans belong to the homo-sapien species. Australopithecus afarensis, known as the first species that lived millions of years ago prior to the existence of homo- sapiens, were known to primarily consume fruit. They were not a part of the cooking era and only consumed raw foods before becoming extinct approximately 1.5 to 3 million years ago (the exact timeframe is unknown). Discovering the Australopithecus diet during that time suggests that a fruitarian lifestyle is healthy and manageable.

The argument healthcare professionals make is the biological differences. Aside from the fact that Australopithecus had an upright posture with a much similar body frame, they have a different physiology compared to humans today. These differences raise concerns about whether we should imitate their diet. Additionally, climate change tends to play a major role in our needs to survive, so most professionals aren't too hyped about what history suggests.

When it comes to the human diet or any species for that matter, it's all about what the digestive system can handle. Considering Australopithecus had a much larger digestive tract, it's advised to avoid comparing modern-day human needs to those of Australopithecus. Humans today are living in different climates with access to fruits and veggies (hybrid foods) that didn't exist millions of years ago. We only consume what we have access to, and a large percentage of that is genetically modified foods. Even an attempt to mimic Australopithecus diet can get very expensive (organic foods) and hard to access depending on where you live.

I have my own questions about fruitarianism, but not as many questions as I have about what historical information suggests that we are meat eaters. In fact, we have no biological similarities to animals nor has the history of human meat eaters shown health benefits of adopting this diet. Animal products cannot be consumed raw or consumed over a long period of time without becoming a major threat to a person's overall health. Raw milk and raw meat are not designed to be processed by the human body. The human diet has evolved into something entirely different even more so after the cooking era began. The human brain became larger and the digestive tract became smaller. When meat was introduced to the human diet, it changed everything we knew about survival without it.

Partially Raw Diet

A partially raw diet is a safe approach for people who want to reap the benefits of a raw diet. A fruitarian diet is underrated; however, it is a high-risk approach when it's not done properly. Refraining from this approach is understandable and probably the best for individuals who are new to dieting. A partially raw diet is gaining popularity at an increasing rate and is often practiced for the sole purpose of detoxing. If you're unfamiliar with a partially raw diet, it's when you only consume raw foods for a certain period of time each day. It's less restrictive and flexible to your daily schedule so you have the luxury of deciding when and how you want to approach it. The most common practice is raw 'til 4. This means you only consume raw foods until 4 pm each day. Depending on your schedule and when you feel the hungriest, you may want to practice the opposite, raw after 4. If a daily detox is your goal, consuming fruit during raw hours would be more helpful since fruit doesn't require much to digest.

There are a few people who prefer fruit only in an effort to cause less harm to plants. None of this is mandatory, and whatever you decide to eat during your raw hours is at your own discretion. Most vegetables such as cabbage, artichoke, greens, and celery are particularly hard to digest and are better consumed when cooked.

I attempted the raw 'til 4 approach and it was a horrible experience for me. If this is not convenient for you, as it wasn't for me, I highly recommend raw after 4 pm. This worked better for me because I was only consuming fruit during my raw hours and fasting right after (sleeping) for the next 8-10 hours. I would feel so refreshed the next morning that I would wake up dreading the feeling of breaking my fast. I enjoyed the feeling of not having anything heavy in my stomach. My intention initially was to do it temporarily, but after I began to see improvement in my digestive health, I knew it was becoming more of a lifestyle change.

After a few months of practicing a partially raw diet, my schedule changed and I became busier throughout the day. Everything I tried seemed inconvenient. I tried the raw until 4 pm and that didn't work out. I went back to my old eating schedule which was eating healthy foods/cooked foods throughout the day. Now that I have balance between work and being a full-time mom, I managed to figure out a way to incorporate fasting back into my daily schedule. Whatever I start my day off eating (cooked or raw) is what I would eat until 4 pm. After 4 pm, would be the opposite. I know it sounds strange, but as I mentioned, my diet is tailored to my needs.

You have the option to modify your diet at any given time. Don't be afraid to change the rules and tweak it to your liking. Nothing about dieting is perfect. Ultimately it's about discovering your own needs and what is most convenient for you.

Digestive Health

Never underestimate the damage that a bad digestive system can cause. Stomach pain, bloating, vomiting, and gas are all symptoms of a bad digestive system. If you've experienced these symptoms, try treating your gut first before thinking you have a terminal disease. Gas and bloating are considered mild effects compared to serious health conditions such as IBS (irritable bowel syndrome), cancer, lactose intolerance, gastric ulcers, and more. What I've found to be more common these days is IBS. I've had a few conversations with people struggling with IBS to the extent that they have to avoid certain healthy foods due to their growing intolerance. This is unfortunate and an awful way to live. What makes me cringe about this is that most people I know with this condition continue to eat the same bad diet that led to their IBS. Instead of making a complete lifestyle change to heal properly, they carry on with life only avoiding foods that cause them to become symptomatic.

For those who are opposed to fruitarianism or fasting, those approaches may help you to reverse your condition. Diseases only thrive in environments that are toxic. If you are eating a bad diet that's ultra-processed over a long period of time, eventually it will lead to conditions such as IBS. Eating foods that don't support digestive health will lead to complications. Your gut makes up 75%-80% of your immune system. If your gut is not functioning properly, you can rest assured that your immune system is not at its best. Your immune system has a close relationship with your digestive system to such a high extent that if you're suffering from any serious health issues anywhere in the body, you MUST start with healing your gut first. Good gut health is the key to reversing any disease caused by a bad diet.

A healthy functioning digestive system can prevent a lot of diseases; however, some illnesses are not caused by the food we eat. I want to make that part clear because while the diet is the leading cause of diseases, it is not the only cause. For example, Lyme disease (LD) is not caused by a bad diet but can manifest quickly in a toxic body. Even when the cause of an illness is unrelated to your diet, the challenges you face after being exposed to it is totally up to the internal environment you create. As I stated before, diseases are only able to thrive in a toxic environment.

You may be in the best health of your life, but don't take advantage of your good health. It's your shield for protection against outside invaders. It's almost like getting life insurance at the age of 20. You don't plan to die anytime soon but you still see fit to get covered in the event of that happening. Sometimes we get so comfortable with feeling well that we forget the discomfort of physical and mental pain. We continue to feed our addiction to certain foods, not realizing it's only a matter of time before we're hit with the ramifications of our actions. A clean diet should be necessary like sleep. If you lose too many hours/days of sleep, you can expect a physical, behavioral, and mental change. I know our body forces us to sleep and it's not really a decision we make, but our body is just as symptomatic when it's overwhelmed with junk.

In spite of being symptomatic, most people still feed the beast of addiction. Never allow your health to take a backseat on your journey of life.

In Conclusion (Part 2) . . .

Part 2 covers the nutritional value in the food we eat and how to stabilize the body's chemistry. Veganism is known for its unattractive labels but there are positive labels that are more appealing. Some are associated with peace, love, and happiness, but those could be misleading. Engaging in other practices in addition to veganism can make those labels fitting for your desired lifestyle since some practices extend beyond the fork.

Expanding your knowledge on nutrient-dense food cultivates healthy physical awareness. It allows you to become in tune with your body and its unique physical needs. Preventing dietary deprivation allows you to escape common fad diets. This happens when you incorporate more foods for volume. The goal is to identify foods in your diet that have little to no nutrients and replace them with foods that are healthy and fulfilling. This sometimes requires you to reduce or eliminate the calories you drink. What you drink is just as important as what you eat. Drinking more water throughout the day keeps your body hydrated and helps the kidney to flush out excess glucose (sugar). It's also a way to buy back wasted calories.

The foundation of any change is mental strength. Don't let the outside world discourage you in believing that certain practices such as fasting, exercising, or mediating are a waste of time. Every journey to success starts with your thinking. Make the decision to get well and fight until you get there. If you can't believe in the power of the process then you won't achieve it. Always keep in mind we are all unique and what works for you may not work for someone else. Be your own example.

Part Three

How To Find The Balance

Chapter 7

The Almighty Vegan Fight

"As you live more mindfully, you eat more mindfully."
~ Lani Muelrath

S ociety has grown sensitive to issues that have resulted in suicide, murder, and serious cases of depression. We've seen a lot of shootings and hate crimes over the years. The core of these incidents spiraled from prejudices, bullying, and public assassination of a person's character. The victims are usually targets because of their personal preference and uncontrollable circumstances such as physical attraction to the same sex, poverty, or race. Most perpetrators are sexist, racist, homophobic/transphobic, or privileged adults/children with little desire to function among those who live differently. Living in this day and time, past transgressions that have gone unspoken are now being publicized on major social platforms causing people to become victims of their past. We no longer have to watch the news or go hunting for information on what's happening in the world because it's thrown in our face every day. You'd have to put in more effort to avoid the news as opposed to hunting for it. The reoccurrence and severity of these situations involve violence against our siblings, friends, and classmates. Being aware of the pain inflicted on families caused by self-serving individuals has increased my intolerance for any form of violence.

Using our voice as a tool to improve our land and protect the animals we share it with is a voice of power. This voice does not serve the same purpose when meaningless messages are sent to the people we wish to recruit. It welcomes negative energy and blocks the message we stand behind. We need to know that the control resides within us in our responses and our approach to the issues we wish to resolve. There is relief in knowing things aren't as bad as they were, but things could be better than they are. We promote the idea that words don't hurt, but in actuality words can hurt more than physical wounds. We have the power to encourage people to change their lives for the better. Let's not be oblivious to our power to discourage people at the same magnitude.

It's not uncommon for people to avoid lifestyles that are challenging especially when the consequence of shying away doesn't bother them. Life is nothing more than a journey. We have little control over what happens to us, but we all have power and control over our reaction and creation of new circumstances. Being kind and respectful should be basic human qualities. Our words are capable of changing someone's life for the better or ruining it for the worse. It doesn't matter how ineffective you feel about making a difference. The fact is your words and actions will always mean something to someone. Your words could mean nothing to me and the world to someone else. People are being attacked daily for their decision to promote certain movements or speak out on certain issues. To change the attitude and the lives of others we'd like to influence, we need to understand the power of our voice and its ability to change things on both ends of the spectrum.

Most acts of violence are handled by our legal system, but the punishment is temporary. The reputation and labels placed on the community of people they represent is tainted indefinitely. We see it happen all the time with Muslims being labeled as terrorists and Catholic priests being labeled as pedophiles. It's unfair, but the power of anyone's actions that's associated with a community of people is affected. The image of that community is what the world sees, not the reputation of one or two individuals.

Veganism is at the peak of its breakthrough. It has become more attractive today than ever before. Companies such as KFC and Burger King are embracing the movement by offering cruelty-free alternatives. I get filled with joy whenever I run across news that a fast food restaurant is launching meat alternatives. I get excited about the recognition of the movement, but I must admit I don't feel a sense of liberation. If you haven't noticed yet, I take pride in guiding others to improve their health. I am not an advocate for companies promoting the idea of meat alternatives being a healthier food option. It's not a purposeless act and a huge step towards liberating our animals and protecting our land, but humans are dying off quickly as we create new ultra-processed food options that are easily accessible, cheap, and convenient.

Putting an End to Bullying

Once we develop a passion for something, we allow our emotions to take full control. In some areas it could be beneficial, but with veganism there's a thin line. The tactics used by members of the vegan community to sway others to transition is borderline bullying. To witness this behavior from adults is disturbing because we've gained enough experience in life to know we cannot control the lives of others with aggression. We have a better chance at making a difference with respect than we do with bullying. My passion to make a difference stems from my love and empathy for people. I find that bullying only leads to rebellion.

As a woman who stands proudly as a vegan, you'd be surprised at what I don't stand for. I do not support PETA, *People for the Ethical Treatment of Animals*. I found their behavior towards Kim Kardashian to be unacceptable and inconsiderate. Their public statement on this incident never suggested their disapproval, but insinuated that this behavior is the consequence of making bad decisions.

The Kim Kardashian attack is a story that made headlines. A woman named Christina Cho (later identified as a PETA member) attacked Kim by pouring a bag of flour on her while on the red carpet for an event. Although PETA denied their involvement with the incident, they had no problem speaking out about what they thought of the situation.

> "PETA has tried everything from polite letters to public protests, but Kim Kardashian has not been moved by the news that animals are beaten, electrocuted, and even skinned alive for real fur garments. Whoever threw that flour may reach her when our polite appeals did not."

Anyone who doesn't find this statement unacceptable is a part of the problem. PETA was very supportive of the attacker after the incident, although they claimed to have no involvement. If Kim didn't feel humiliated enough from being flour-bombed, PETA proceeded with another act of harassment. They posted an antagonizing billboard of two foxes with a caption that stated "Kim: These babies miss their mother. IS SHE ON YOUR BACK?" as if Kim is the only person in the world who wears fur. Even reflecting on this makes me angry because this is the epitome of bullying and harassment. To make matters worse, they used her popularity and fame to get recognition despite the humiliation and disapproval of Kim and her family. I will never support PETA because violence is never acceptable and I don't stand for organizations that are pro-bullying when it's an act that pushes their agenda.

Most vegans and animal activists today were not born vegans. We all ate meat and dairy products at least once or twice in our lives. I understand how we've grown to become passionate about our beliefs, but we cannot act oblivious to how we lived prior to our lifestyle change. If someone attacked or flour bombed us while being publicly humiliated for our legal right and preference to consume meat, we would be furious. I do not place all the blame on the vegan community or PETA supporters, but as late rapper Biggie Smalls stated "We can't change the world unless we change ourselves." Let's focus on us as a vegan community and determine how we can become a positive representation of what we believe. Violence is the easiest most ignorant way to get someone's attention. That's how we want to be remembered? I don't want my daughter to grow up seeing how I aggressively approached and attacked anyone who chose to live a different lifestyle than ours. This is tough love from one fellow vegan to another that we must change our approach.

If you are out protesting or filming to create a documentary in support of your non-profit organization for the mistreatment of animals, you are doing a great service for the vegan community. There are non-profit organizations such as Animal Liberation Front (ALF), Mercy for Animals and Last Chance for Animals that are actively putting an end to animal cruelty. I support the common cause we all share, but I am very selective about what I choose to represent. What I am finding is how often members of these organizations are being arrested for theft (stealing animals off farmers' property) and violence. Some members of these organizations have become clever in their approach to serving the community. For example, Direct Action Everywhere is a new group with Animal Liberation that was found in 2013. James Warren, member of Direct Action Everywhere, spoke out against a farmer named Jason Parravicini after a video surfaced of the farmer shooting in the air as a warning to James and his colleagues. After the video went viral, James proclaimed to be nonviolent and innocent during the acrimonious exchange. I thought this was odd so I dug a little deeper to see what really transpired. After gathering more information on the incident, I was able to see why things escalated so quickly. James and his colleagues showed up outside of Jason's farm/property unannounced to record the activity on Jason's farm. Furious as anyone would be, Jason demanded that they leave; they refused. The fight was destined to take place.

This story made headlines and everyone gave their biased opinion on the incident. Both James and Jason spoke out on the incident. Based on the story they both shared, James and his colleagues were nonviolent; however, the tactic used was antagonizing. The farmer should've handled the situation in a nonviolent manner, but James also knew it was an antagonizing approach to show up just outside someone's farm to film activity on their property without permission. To intentionally provoke someone is a form of bullying even if it's not an illegal offense. There are animal advocates who have done great work in the community without being antagonistic, disrespectful, or violent. Being stuck in the game of checkers is only a social distraction. Real strategists make real changes as if it's a game of chess. Delayed gratification is commonly understood and respected among strategists. Taking extreme measures to create the right timing for something to happen does nothing for our community.

The battle didn't begin or end with James and Jason. Several other members of the same group were arrested for stealing turkeys and chickens that were being raised by farmers. As many non-profit (animal activists') organizations claim to not condone violence, they take pride in the behavior of their members. The list of the unlawful acts made by these members continues to happen. Hearing about violence from people in a community I support upsets me. I don't agree with the lifestyle of the people in my community or family members in reference to their diet, but I respect their decision and free will to eat and live the life they desire. Being passionate about something is one thing, but being vindictive, malicious, spiteful, violent, and disrespectful is another. Nothing about what occurred that day was peaceful or influential. For animal activists to have so much experience on how past situations escalated, they had to know their approach was antagonizing. It only provokes those currently using animal products for food and luxury items to be even more rebellious and violent in retaliation to blatant disrespect. The vegan community does not agree with the world's attitude about the mistreatment of our animals, but we have to be mindful that it's not illegal. It's their lawful right to kill animals for food, makeup, clothing, and whatever else they choose to use it for.

Don't jeopardize future opportunities and time away from your family by getting arrested and charged for a cause that you made even harder for people to gravitate towards. Invading someone's privacy or personal space isn't a strategic move or persuasive in any way. Who learns from violence? Even with Kim getting flour-bombed on the red carpet, it was noble of her not to file charges. If she had filed charges against her assailant, she would have left that situation for her legal team to handle and carried on with her life. You would then have a woman in jail dealing with the ramifications of her actions while Kim wore whatever it is that she wanted. It seems quite pointless when you put it into perspective. What is gained from making your life difficult in an effort to expose someone else in front of people who live the same life and may have no intentions on transitioning? If Kim had any thoughts of one day becoming an advocate for animal rights like her sister Khloe who was formerly a PETA supporter, that idea probably faded away quickly in result of this one extreme incident.

What the World Really Sees

Getting feedback from non-vegans helped me identify where we need improvement. People often have their guard up once they discover I'm vegan, but I empathize with them and make them feel comfortable. I want them to be able to talk with me because I know how it feels to be on the other side. I take pride in being an example of what veganism is truly about. The feedback I receive helps me understand why we continue to have these problems today after years of seeing where our actions have led us.

I was on Instagram one day when I ran across a video of the "Insta-famous" Brittany Renner expressing her thoughts about vegans. She first made a joke about the lifestyle but proceeded with something that caught my attention. She said "I like poking fun of vegans because you guys move like a cult and it fascinates me. I feel like sometimes the message is lost in the style of recruiting." It was one of those unexpected eureka moments where all my presumptions were confirmed. She was making a joke and probably didn't think much of it, but that captivating statement, "the message is sometimes lost in the style of recruiting" perfectly articulates how most non-vegans feel. What I took from that is people believe we have no boundaries in our approach. We are known to take action with violence, antagonism, and invasion of privacy to relay a message that's overshadowed by our absence of nobility.

Addiction

I empathize with non-vegans only because of my own struggles and addictions. I was unaware of my addictions until I attempted to make a change. Making the decision to take better care of myself was the easy part. I focused on the basic approach like eliminating sugar, fried foods, and snacks from my diet. I thought eliminating sugar would be unchallenging considering my dislike for candy and my love for salty treats (chips, salty nuts, etc.).

Sugar contributes a lot to how our food tastes. Corn bread, canned corn, BBQ sauce, peanut butter, and baked beans were foods I ate regularly. I didn't think of the sugar content that contributed to the taste that attracted me in the first place. It wasn't until I started reading food labels that I realized the struggle was real. The sugar-free versions were horrible. I no longer craved BBQ sauce, peanut butter, or baked beans because it was the sugar that made them tasteful and addictive. Eliminating the sugar from my favorite foods and sauces obliterated my interest. I would relapse every other week to the point of becoming a part of the yo-yo dieting club. Inconsistency was the only way to describe my diet when fitness became a part of my journey. One day I would be on top of my game following my meal plan, and the next I would binge eat like it was my last meal. My consistency thrived in the area of fitness training. It was my love for fitness that kept me motivated to find a balanced diet. The last thing I wanted to be was counter-productive. It took a few years to find a healthy balance, but I did it.

I was fortunate enough to live in a state where I didn't have family or friends to disrupt my process. I worked from home so I wasn't tempted by company potlucks or Christmas parties where food was the primary focus. It was just me and my one-year-old daughter who was just getting introduced to table food. I had more control over my process than most could say about theirs. I could only imagine what my process would have been if I had family near or if I worked in an office environment where food and snacks were always around. The story I'm sharing now may have turned out a lot different.

I know the advantages I had and yet I still struggled. I don't know if it's my journey or my character that makes me empathetic, but whatever it is I am grateful for it. It's a process and I know from experience that if someone was trying to force something on me that I wasn't ready for I would become rebellious and reciprocate the negative energy that I felt. Anything involving a change in behavior should be something the person views as a pleasant experience. If the light can't be seen at the end of the tunnel because it's blocked by anger, aggression, or bitterness, then as you may expect the outcome will always be the same.

I understand that some animal activists and vegans were born into the lifestyle so it's difficult for them to empathize with others. They only know what they've been taught and if meat or dairy was never introduced to their diet, I can understand why it's viewed as an easy task for anyone to do. It seems the only animals that are taken into consideration are animals that we adopt as members of our family such as dogs, cats, hamsters, and rabbits. We don't typically welcome pigs, cows, or chickens into our home.

I named this book The Vegan Fight because it's a fight within. I love animals and I love their role in nature. It's unacceptable to eat animals or use them to evolve in the fashion/cosmetic industry. I don't agree with taking animals from the wilderness and keeping them locked up in a zoo for local amusement. I never liked the zoo and will never take my daughter there because I don't find it amusing at all. I am passionate about our environment, animals, and most importantly human health. Nothing I'm saying justifies the behavior nor does it reflect my level of concern. It has everything to do with my personality and the order in which I believe things should be handled.

Human health is still my primary focus, but as I explained, we can't thrive without advocating the three forces. Our health depends on the conditions of our environment which is directly affected by animal agriculture. When I make a decision to be a part of a movement, I handle it as I would in my personal life. It's never wise to point out the shortcomings of someone or a group of people without addressing our role in the situation. Since I am a part of the vegan community, I chose to address our contribution to the problem.

We're always involved in misunderstandings. We are falsely accused of things that didn't happen and even attacked because of past events. How the situation plays out is based upon the personalities of the people involved. I've had people give me attitude and criticized my way of living without me saying a word. I know that it's their defense mechanism to prepare them for whatever it is they presume I, as a vegan, am going to say or do. There are vegans who just live the lifestyle and could care less about convincing others to do the same. When they are disrespected or attacked because they identify themselves as vegan it becomes personal. Whatever happens after that has nothing to do with the vegan cause and everything to do with someone feeling disrespected. In this scenario neither party may have cared about how the other chose to live. Because one group made assumptions about the other, things escalated quickly. Unfortunately, vegans' involvement in any altercation regarding their way of living promotes the idea that vegans are insensitive.

Nothing can truly prepare you for what may come your way with this lifestyle. You may one day have the craziest story to tell someone else, but make sure that story doesn't end in violence. Our decision to live a certain way is not limited to our diet. We make decisions every day to be a part of something that I'm certain everyone doesn't agree with. It's a part of life and being in an awkward situation where you feel disrespected is inevitable. For the most part, it's a welcoming lifestyle and whether you believe it or not, non-vegans are more interested in learning about the lifestyle than you might think. While they might not necessarily be interested in transitioning, they are interested in becoming more knowledgeable about our lifestyle.

The fight we're having today is the fight within ourselves. We are constantly fighting to control our emotions and addictions. Our way of thinking about what is supposed to happen in our lives and how people must treat us, conflicts with reality. When this occurs, a person may feel overwhelmed with high emotions feeling violated and full of rage. It's an inner disturbance that takes away a person's peace and sense of understanding. We live in a society where people seek to demand a certain type of behavior from others. Situations that escalate quickly are not inevitable. This is not to say our thoughts are wrong and things shouldn't be the way we imagine, but it's based on how things really are. We should be passionate enough about something that it arouses different emotions. That's what helps us discover our purpose in life and service to others. The main purpose in life is to identify a problem that you'd like to solve and set out to make a change.

In order to make a change we must be emotionally involved to some extent; however, our thoughts and emotions should not be so powerful that we forget the reality of things. If Martin Luther King, Jr. or Rosa Parks handled their beliefs with aggression or violence, we wouldn't know who they are today. More than likely, King and Parks would have been murdered, served years in prison, or lost their voice before they gained a level of recognition to impact the world. Building their platform required patience, commitment, optimism, and understanding. King discussed his vision for the future in his 1953 speech,

"I Have A Dream." While he had high hopes of school integration, fair treatment, and equality, he knew and respected the time he was living in and emphasized the demand for a nonviolent movement from his followers. He knew how violence could affect the message he wanted to share and proceeded on his journey with that in mind.

While the messages are different, the outcome is similar. They've experienced more unfair treatment and disrespect than we could imagine in this day and time. Back then, there were no lies to cover your true feelings or pretending not to be a racist when you really were. People were very clear about their thoughts and acted in a manner in which they wanted towards African Americans. As things began to change and we stepped in a time where the disabled, homosexuals, African Americans, etc. found a voice and demanded respect and fair treatment, that was the beginning of a demanding society.

I feel relieved at how many people I've touched and how I motivated them to do the research about how to live a sustainable vegan lifestyle. Meat eaters rarely deny that veganism has its benefits for human health and for the health of our environment. They know it's a healthier way of living and how it could change the world if we all become more mindful of the things we decide to consume. In a world full of disappointment, wickedness, betrayal, and disloyalty, people want to be able to have at least one guaranteed pleasurable moment every day. Eating is something people look forward to throughout the day whether it's their lunch break at work to reboot them with joy or dinner in the evening after a hard day of work and a busy schedule with the kids. The last thing on a person's mind during the day is whether the food they are eating for lunch or dinner is good for the environment or their health. They don't care about any of that, especially when much of the world is doing the same thing.

Accept What You Can't Change

This will be tough for my animal lovers, but it must be said. There are people you CANNOT change. They will die with a piece of chicken in their mouth and that's just the reality of it. You can fight with them, argue with them, and threaten them, but that will not change how they feel or what choices they'll make in the future. They are content with accepting the consequences of eating animal products including the damage to our environment, the mistreatment of our animals, and their increased susceptibility to diseases. Since meat-eaters and vegans are susceptible to the same diseases according on their diet, it doesn't cause much concern for meat-eaters. Some people just don't desire to change at all. Let's focus on the people we do have access to who are willing to learn about the lifestyle.

How to Handle a Lost Cause

If you're an active animal activist I'm sure you've experienced a few lost causes from people working in the animal agriculture. Some people are not interested in changing their mind set. There are people in the cemetery today who took childhood pain, stubbornness, and bad habits with them. It's vital that we accept that there are people we won't be able to change. We should not proceed with aggression or demand them to change because we'll fail every time. Instead, we should identify when it's a lost cause and move on to encourage those who are open to change. There's truth in the serenity prayer: "God grant me the serenity to accept the things I cannot change; courage to change the things I can; and the wisdom to know the difference." This applies to every aspect of life whether you believe in God or not. Keeping this in mind will help mitigate some of the fights and battles you face along your journey.

The vegan fight isn't physical or demanding. We can continue to reach people from all walks of life to make a difference in the world. How we treat others is a direct reflection of how we feel about ourselves. The tone we set today will impact future generations that will be influenced by our fight today.

Chapter 8

The Power of Unity

"Our unity is our strength and diversity is our power."
~ Kamala Harris

U nity is a bond that thrives through truth and purpose. Fighting over our differences is based on our interpretation of the facts. Dr. Tony Evans once stated "truth is bigger than facts." The damage a meat-based/dairy-based diet can cause is not a mystery to non-vegans. In some instances, they would tell you the facts so they could avoid the topic of why there are a million reasons to transition. Society is willing and ready to accept the facts, but the truth appears to be too much to handle. The truth forces us to address issues from our own experiences in life and reality, whereas facts don't belong to a particular person or experience, and can be false based on our interpretation of the factual information. The truth is already interpreted. When it comes to an animal-based diet, we see its contribution to global warming, animal injustice, and the damage to human health; but that's just facts. The truth is buried within us all and hides from the world like the master of disguise.

Knowing our exposure to diseases is easy to accept, but what challenges us is acknowledging the impact. Low self-esteem and lack of confidence are things that force us to face the foundation of our truths. We hide the pain we feel from losing a loved one to diabetes, heart disease, and other diseases that are terminal, but we continue to live a life that led to their demise. We act surprised when diseases cripple our loved ones, but we internalize our feelings and move on. We may act unbothered, but nothing cause an emotional disturbance more than the silent cries underneath our mask when we can't save our own children from depression as a result of being teased or bullied for being overweight. Truth resides in areas we hide. There's nothing friendly or soothing about it. It's ruthless and the hardest pill to swallow and yet, it's the only thing that liberates us.

Unity only exists when there is power in the purpose. Purpose is acknowledging with truth where we maintain clarity on where we're trying to go. This goes back to Brittany Renner's statement: we cannot operate like a cult with the expectation of attracting people to veganism. We cannot encourage people to transition, and then criticize them for failing to follow all the rules. It's counterproductive behavior that leads to more confusion as we attempt to impact future generations. Truth and purpose live outside our personal admirations, beliefs, and preferences. Creating unity is about having a receptive attitude with an ability to have an open dialogue without judgment. Unity based on a common bond is easy; creating a bond with someone who doesn't share your passion is the real challenge. It forces you to respect the thoughts and opinions of others based on the power of a diverse perspective. Have you ever wondered how two people with nothing in common become friends or business partners? It's not because they agree on everything, it's because of their thirst for objectiveness from various perspectives.

Missing opportunities to impact lives due to our twisted idea that unity is about shared emotions depletes our strength and creates a loss of momentum. Everyone wants to feel like they belong even when they don't believe it themselves. We strive to be a part of something that's bigger than ourselves in an area that we've neglected for so many years. Although people might not express their interests out loud, they might be interested. Every living being has a story. The influential aspect behind each story is uniquely aligned for each and every one of our lives. What we consider as normal is whatever environment and group of people we invite into our thoughts and hearts. As cliché as it sounds, we are the product of our environment; we are the product of the energy we welcome.

Imagine being known as a charismatic, upbeat group of people that captivates the world with charm. People would gravitate towards us on the basis of our reputation. One thing we all have in common is our desire for peace. During my college days, I would eat at Chick-fil-A just for good customer service. I could be craving something from Wendy's or McDonald's, but my desire for a pleasant experience I could rely on was more important to me than anything else. They always exceeded my expectations and I could always rely on them to put my sauce in the bag without having to ask twice or be disappointed because they forgot. Nothing compares to Chick-fil-A's impressive customer service. I know this example is a bad comparison considering our fight to promote a cruelty-free lifestyle, but the point is to highlight their strategic approach. They weren't trying to come up with new ways to make a chicken sandwich or launch something out of their lane like tacos; their aim was to attract people to the experience.

Even with a diverse staff, Chick-fil-A managed to create a system that effectively communicates to a diverse group people on how to perform according to the company's vision. Do you know how difficult that is to do? To have influence on a level that encourages people to perform in a manner that executes your vision? That could only happen through unity. Whatever training is conducted or information communicated to their new hires, it's meticulously formulated to instill an attitude that eventually touches the world in a compassionate way.

Unity is Our Strength

Strength is something we think we all have until it's put to the test. Any effort in being effective in life comes with a level of discomfort. This could range from simple fears with a little anxiety, to sadness and extreme rage. We all have our triggers as vegans. My biggest trigger is being profiled because of my lifestyle as a vegan. I like for people to get to know me first before presuming my character, but I'm also aware of the labels forced on the vegan lifestyle so my response is never defensive. People who transition for health purposes aren't typically bothered by the lifestyle of others. We aren't invested in people who don't desire to change. We accept them for who they are and continue to help those who are ready. On the other hand, vegans who transition for animal rights are invested to the fullest extent. They want to reach the unreachable, even when they know the outcome won't be in their favor.

I had a friend a few years ago who would always ask me to choose the restaurant when we would go out to eat. One day, I asked her to choose because I was indecisive. She hesitated and started to name vegan restaurants. I told her I didn't have a problem eating at a non-vegan restaurant if that's what she wanted. I wasn't starving that day, so I was ok with ordering a salad. She got quiet for a moment thinking of things to say and then named a vegan restaurant. I didn't want to press the issue because I didn't want to make things awkward. I obliged and we ate at one of my favorite vegan restaurants in Atlanta, Georgia, Go Vegan. It wasn't until our eighth month of friendship that

I asked her if she was vegan. I never saw her eat meat or dairy products and couldn't take another eight months in suspense. I just blurted out one day in mid-conversation, "Are you vegan?" The question was random so I'm certain she was taken back. She responded quickly with "Heck no! I would never give up meat or milk!" I was in total shock.

I wasn't shocked because I expected her to be vegan. I was shocked because she hid that part of her life from me. I had to pry because for someone to love meat so much I figured I would know as her friend of eight months. After overwhelming her with questions, she had no desire to be interrogated any longer, so she told me her food choices are different around me to avoid offending me. She proceeded to say, "I don't want my diet to affect our friendship or make you uncomfortable to where you don't want to eat out or hang out with me anymore." I was in utter disbelief to the point that I don't believe I responded to her immediately. I had to process what she said and reflect on all the times she pretended to want vegan food when she really didn't. I appreciated the act of respect but I felt awful.

The first thought I had was, "Did she enjoy the food we ate or was that a lie?" I felt like I made her feel uncomfortable our entire friendship. I wondered if the reputation of the vegan community made her feel it was necessary to hide her lifestyle. How could I sit and stuff my face with food without thinking once if she enjoyed any of the food she ordered? How could I not ask if she was vegan? I felt inconsiderate for a while after discovering her feelings but needless to say, I went back to her and made it very clear where I stand as a vegan and as a friend. I respected her lifestyle and diet as she did with mine. Yes, I would have loved for her to be vegan. However, whatever life choices she wanted to make I was prepared to respect and support her. Her dietary choices didn't stand a chance in ruining our friendship.

I was able to see how people perceived me and my personality based on my diet. It was an eye-opening experience. How can we make a change when we can't face the problem head on or function in a non-vegan environment? To make a difference requires us to step outside our comfort zone. To engage with people who are not vegans and allow them to comfortably express themselves without feeling judged. Although we may not agree with how they choose to fulfill their hunger, we can demonstrate our patience and willingness to be there whenever they're ready to take that first step.

Sometimes you find yourself having to put your feelings aside for a greater good. Think about how many people work alongside Donald Trump yet disagree with his decisions. He offends people daily with his Twitter rants, but you don't see his constituents resigning or compromising their positions because of their dislike for him. Their objective is to make a difference. When you avoid the feeling of being uncomfortable, you avoid making a change. Your head should be as high as it would be if everyone agreed with you. Your smile should be as warming as it would be if everything turned out in your favor. Face the discomfort head on to make a change. Make respect a priority when faced with opposition. CEOs, VPs, etc. don't get paid the big bucks doing the least amount of work because they're smart. They were hired and paid the big bucks to handle opposition. They are evaluated based on their ability to manage.

Vibrating on a High Frequency

Negative energy comes without warning. It creeps in with a change of thoughts, feelings, and attitude. Excessive negative thinking, blaming others for your feelings and a number of bad relationships are all symptoms of an emerging decline in frequency. Negativity contaminates everything you encounter and causes you to think that you aren't the problem. The common denominator stares at you in the mirror every chance it gets, but you ignore it. Operating at a higher frequency requires intense self-evaluation mentally, spiritually, and emotionally. It affects your attitude towards others, your ability to achieve your goals, and your likelihood to make a difference in the world. Finding peace of mind in this wicked world is imperative. That doesn't make you weak or an advocate for things you find unacceptable. That makes you aligned and able to function in environments, to engage in conversations that don't fit into your thoughts of reality.

How I Handle Discomfort

I enjoy yoga for various reasons. A peace of mind is the priority, but to challenge myself physically strengthens my self-control. Yin yoga has allowed me to reach new measures since I am required to hold uncomfortable positions over an extended period of time. In the beginning it felt like torture, but over time I became obsessed with my ability to see it through. Yoga has challenged me in all areas of life to continue, even when I feel like I'm losing control. Having self-discipline requires practice. The urge to say something or do something is so powerful that it sometimes feels like an addiction. It's not always easy to engage in a conversation with someone who has made up their mind to be misunderstood or ignorant. Since the beginning of time, truth rarely resulted in victory. Fighting for the truth to be accepted is much more difficult than fighting for a lie to be heard and accepted.

Increasing your vibration involves focusing on the energy you put out. What are your thoughts? What makes you react in a way that's not conducive to what you're trying to accomplish? Why isn't your style of productivity working for you? I've seen animal activists work day in and day out with little to no success in making a difference. When it comes to their interaction with people who don't abide by their living standard, there's chaos. This is the trouble area where most people vibration declines drastically. The energy shifts from positive to negative almost instantly. All sense of understanding, respect, and kindness are no longer contributing factors in their approach to rectify the problem. In order to vibrate at a high frequency to create the unity we aim for, we must operate in uncomfortable situations. I struggled with this in my personal life and was reminded time after time that my anger and blatant disrespect were not conducive to what I was trying to accomplish in the situation.

Let's revert back to PETA versus Kim Kardashian. There's so much to learn from their statements on the attack that everything about it was distasteful. After Khloe made her public statement to no longer support the organization, PETA wasted no time to give their rebuttal:

> "We appreciate that Khloe will remain on the animals' side by not wearing fur, that's what counts. If one of our volunteers is responsible, it doesn't alter the fact that no animal deserves to be electrocuted, shot, or poisoned for a bit of fur clothing. Khloe is just defending her sister. We just wish she also had more influence on her sister."

PETA Spokesperson

Considering that a big part of unity is truth, this situation was solely about being selective to the facts and responding. PETA knew that what happened to Kim was wrong, but since we are not operating in truth, they decided to deflect the media's attention by focusing on animal rights. If I were the spokesperson for PETA I would have started with an apology on behalf of our volunteer to ensure the public knew that we do not condone that type of behavior to push our agenda. Then I would have proceeded to expose the suffering of animals and how their welfare should be taken into consideration. Do you see the difference between the two approaches?

Kim didn't kill the animal herself; she purchased the fur like a million other people. The message PETA sent was that they condone violence against those who are not moved by their protests and polite letters. Sounds to me like they believed she deserved it. Where is the respect in that? There's no unity when we circumvent the truth or make statements that suggest we condone violence. I'm passionate about this because the people we attack are the same people we are trying to influence. When we identify a lost cause we proceed with violence. It's almost like saying since we can't change you; we have nothing to lose by hurting you, disrespecting you, or wishing the worst for you. That's insane to me. Animal lives are not the only lives that matter. In my world, all lives matter so I proceed with dignity and respect.

Sending out positive energy and vibration allows me to reach people I had no clue cared or were interested after considering our first encounter and writing them off as a lost cause. We sometimes try to force things or create situations that are not aligned with the proper chain of events. All things come together at the right time, not on our time. A friend of mine once mentioned how Richard Pryor would have never succeeded in this day and time as a stand-up comedian. I laughed because I knew exactly why he said that. We evolved with time and we've become more cautious about our responses to certain issues or topics. I hear more public apologies today than I've heard during my childhood/teenage years. Richard Pryor was known as one of the most uncensored comedians ever. He was successful in his time, but without a doubt he would have failed miserably if he approached comedy the same way today. Kevin Hart has to be at least in the top 5 comedians who try to be politically correct. Even with his fame and fortune, he still received backlash from a tweet he posted over six years ago. The tweet resurfaced after he accepted the offer as a host for the Oscars.

The controversy surrounding the tweet led to Kevin's decision to later decline the offer.

This is just a glimpse of how quickly things changed from Richard Pryor's time to Kevin Hart's time. What appears to be acceptable today by society maybe unacceptable tomorrow. The only thing that remains constant is the results we get when using violence and operating on a lower frequency. Without unity, we'll only repeat history as we have for the past couple of decades. Nothing will change and everyone will still eat meat and wear fur and whatever else they feel is pleasing to them.

Digging Deeper in the Truth

Animal activists have long been identified as a movement that serves white America. For many years, animal activists have been fighting for the rights of our animals while ignoring the mistreatment of black America. To be quite honest, animals were treated better than blacks for many years. Blacks weren't getting murdered for human consumption or skinned for boots. They were murdered because of the color of their skin. Was this forgotten or are the lives of people of color unimportant? In early years, vegans and animal activists were predominantly white (middle class and upper class). A few were willing to lose their life and freedom to protect our animals, but refused to do the same for their own species. Although the treatment of African Americans has improved over the years, we are still facing racial prejudices.

In April 2015, an unarmed black man named Walter Scott was murdered by a white cop named Michael Slager. Although justice was served in this case, black America mourned his tragic death. As expected, white America rarely focuses on the brutal mistreatment of African Americans or views it as news-worthy, but that's not the alarming part with this particular incident. What's alarming about this is just three months after Walter was gunned down, white America was in a state of devastation over the death of Cecil the Lion. I don't claim to be the brightest person, but I sure wondered where the energy was when Walter was murdered.

The point is to acknowledge peoples' need to be understood and cared for. If they feel their life is unimportant to you, then it's a strong possibility they won't support your beliefs or desire to listen to anything you have to say. Unity is supporting all races and acknowledging the rights of the human race. This is not just about black America; it's about equal rights for all. Once we learn to respect and serve our own kind (humankind), then we'll be able to reach people to reciprocate the respect and concern even if they don't necessarily desire to. They will listen because we listened.

Chapter 9

Birth Our Future

"Change the way you look at things and the things you look at change."
~ Wayne W. Dyer

The decisions we make today will affect tomorrow either positively or negativity. History is forever written and rarely forgotten. You can capitalize on it by owning it and creating new memories in the minds of target audiences, or you can perpetuate past behavior because history is not the centerpiece of your thinking. Whatever you do, please note that what matters today is what can be done to improve tomorrow. How we imagine the future and the change we desire to see should coincide with our behavior, even when change appears impossible. Changing the future depends upon our actions and behavior but mainly our attitude. Our ideas and behavior are conditioned to how things are today, but that may be a downfall when attempting to make a change. We should walk our path with confidence as if the change we desire has already manifested. Our biggest problem when fighting for a change is becoming discouraged because no one has done what we're aiming to do. Everything that's happening today has once been labeled impossible. Don't be afraid to be the first to do something. Imagine if the Wright brothers had given up on building a flying machine (airplane). At the time of their attempt, no one was successful in creating a flying source of transportation. Because they were able to condition their mind to see new realities, they were able to manifest it and become the first to do it.

Change starts with your imagination. Imagine if everything you've ever imagined was achievable. Now imagine it all being possible at the right time; without force, without verbal or physical altercations, but with consistency, love, and passion. Allow yourself to feel content in the season you're in and to accept that this season may not be your season of manifestation. Even through the emotional rollercoaster of feeling discouraged and defeated, you feel power in embracing the creation of your footprint that will affect future generations. What's the likelihood of everyone giving up meat? What are the odds of it being weird to be a meat eater? The idea of it seems insane today, especially since we've embraced a meat-eating lifestyle for so many years. We have people stepping into entrepreneurship as mukbangers who eat pounds of meat and dairy products for their viewers' amusement. Mukbang videos show people sitting and eating thousands of calories to entertain their ASMR audience. Seafood has become a trend within the mukbang community, but now people are ordering tons of food from fast food restaurants like McDonalds, Popeye's, Fat Burger, and KFC as well as cooking large amounts of meat and other homemade dishes to captivate people all over the world. This is our reality today. Our parents and grandparents would have never imagined this style of entrepreneurship 20 years ago.

Knowing how things change so quickly, how can you believe things will be the same 20 years from now? Look how long slavery lasted. I'm sure that telling someone back then that blacks and whites would one day share the same schools, occupations, voting rights, and career opportunities would probably get you admitted into a mental institution. We have no clue what our work today will do for the future. Even some of the fast food restaurants I've mentioned are adding vegan options to their menu. The impossible burger has become immensely popular over the past year. Although these are baby steps towards what we hope for, it's those steps that matters the most. One way or another, we will find a way to achieve our goals.

When I transitioned, there weren't any fast food vegan options available. I couldn't go through drive thru and pick up a burger on my way to work. I had to prepare my meals or opt for a salad or fries. Things are changing and restaurants are noticing the demand for vegan options. I've been vegan less than six years now and if I'm able to see so much change within a short amount of time, I'm ecstatic to see what could happen in 20 years. Patience is a virtue and if we can understand that, we'll get there in due time.

I know first-hand it's not easy to transition. I'm unsure how long it would have taken me if the body aches didn't step in and completely put a pause on my life. We must be patient with everyone. This is learned behavior, not a decision we had the ability to make at birth. Anyone who holds a leadership position (parent, primary guardian, aunts, uncles, teachers, and doctors) has an impact on the development of future generations. Our message can't be lost in the fight because our behavior speaks louder than our good deeds.

I will never diminish the importance of animal rights, but I do not see the point of diminishing the importance of good health and environmental sustainability. The truth is that not everyone is a fan of animals. Quite frankly, some people dislike that it's a topic of conversation. The mistreatment of animals and the disheartening images thrown in their faces as a tactic to make them feel horrible about eating meat means nothing to them. What these same people may care about is their health or the environment. Although we can't control what they are passionate about, we can control the angle to get their attention on what we want to put an end to.

Our Public Figures Matter

The people who are suffering the wrath of our dislike are public figures. I hate to say it but I believe this is the dumbest approach ever. Public figures have a large social following with a strong fan base. Fans tend to take on views of their favorite artist, social influencer, president, or former president. We can't go around burning bridges because we politely asked them to be an advocate for the vegan movement and they declined. Either give up or keep trying until they give in, but it makes no sense to damage relationships before we can build them. If they aren't moved by our kindness, their kind words about who we are could influence a lot of people to change their diet.

We are living in an impatient time where waiting is not a part of the strategy. Being impatient says a lot about a person. Their better judgment is lost in anger, frustration, anxiety, and unhappiness. The urge to want everything to happen right now is a selfish and ungrateful emotion that blocks future accomplishments. This mentality won't yield long-term results and rarely makes a difference in present time. Protesting and being an advocate for our animals is great, but be wise about it. I can't tell you how many stories I've heard about Jehovah's Witnesses knocking on doors early in the morning upsetting people, but I never heard of them becoming violent or disrespecting the people who turn them away. They get back up the next morning and knock on the same doors as if nothing ever occurred the day prior. That's the mentality one should possess as an advocate for animals.

I want future generations to be inspired by our work. Being kind doesn't cost a thing. Having the power to stand for this movement should include an equal power to refrain from dramatic engagements. One component of maturity is identifying bad decisions and making better ones. This level of maturity prevents people from different backgrounds from thinking human lives are secondary to animal lives. Immigrants are still fighting for their freedom and the freedom of their family members. African Americans are still fighting for fair treatment. If people are still fighting for their freedom and rights as human beings, trying to shift their focus to the importance of animal lives while disregarding theirs is a little insensitive.

Animals have been a source of food long before the past five generations. There's not a person alive today who is primarily responsible for the meat eating evolution. Most times you have to think outside your own understanding and consider the circumstances surrounding today's world of meat eaters. Being understanding doesn't mean you agree with their views; it merely means that you understand the circumstances and difficulties surrounding their life choices. What we are doing is bigger than us. Let's leave our children inspired to stand for something that's more than a cult-like community.

People who refuse to identify themselves as vegan are not avoiding the lifestyle; they are avoiding the negative energy and environment that permeates society. The problem with what we bring is our pattern of aggression. Once a pattern has been identified it's hard to break it. Justifying our immoral acts is just an excuse we give ourselves to act on our personal feelings. When we lack self-control we neglect our purpose and embark on a path of stagnation. The labels can be annoying, especially when they don't apply to you. It can be nerve wracking when you know you don't fit the profile. This only gives others confirmation that nothing about the vegan journey has changed.

Channeling our inner strength through proper evaluation will allow us to conquer all things.

Embrace the Journey to Birth

Birthing a child is an unforgettable experience. From the time of conception to giving birth, you can expect bodily changes along with symptoms to occur during each stage of pregnancy. There are three trimesters in a pregnancy and each trimester has its own specific symptoms that are triggered by fetal development and hormonal changes. As much as women would love to skip all three trimesters to give birth to a bundle of joy, it doesn't work that way so morning sickness to fluttering fetal movements are bitter sweet moments that set the foundation of an unforgettable bond.

Our vision for the future is no different than giving birth to a child. To birth the future, we must endure troubled times that represent the stages of growth and progress. As with any pregnancy, the peaceful option is enjoying the process with the end goal in mind. To some extent we're all aware of the battles that come with setting life-changing milestones. We may not be aware of the severity of the battles or how tragic the encounter, but as women take risks with health challenges and potential birth defects, we know it could be worse than what we imagine.

Knowing the possibilities during pregnancy may overwhelm any woman. Some women may feel so frightened by the idea of having a child that they seek other alternatives like an abortion or adoption. We have this same option with our passion and purpose. We can choose to abort the journey or let someone else live our dream, or fight through the stages while knowing possible detours that may transpire. It's easy to get blinded by the hardships, but as the strength of our passion grows inside of us and gets stronger, we know the return for our investment is worth the fight.

Reaching the end of the third trimester can be more frightening than the pregnancy journey because it's the start of a new fight. Once the baby is fully developed after weeks of growing, it's time to give birth. The birth of a child is the first step into reality that you've completed the first milestone of carrying the child. The day of birth is the day of truth. On that day, we all speculate what could happen while facing the last fight of pregnancy to welcome your child into this world. All we have in that moment as a parent is to hope and wish everything goes well in the delivery room. We reflect on all the healthy steps taken throughout the pregnancy including taking prenatal vitamins, exercising, eating healthy foods, meditating, and relieving stress. In that moment of giving birth you are hoping that you did your best in developing a healthy baby. Before any of that is revealed, the final step is crucial: pushing. Using your last ounce of energy and strength to finally see what has been growing inside of you for the past 40 weeks is the epitome of a bitter sweet moment. Think about the aspiration that's been growing inside of us for years. How that feeling becomes more and more intense as time goes by. That feeling alone is the identifier of our purpose but that growing feeling has stages. Being impregnated with a deep passion to see the world evolve and become compassionate for the environment and non-human lives is more than just a stage in life. It's preparing us to give birth to future generations to manifest our vision.

When a woman finds out she's pregnant, there are changes she must make to adjust to what is expected to come. If she drinks alcohol on the weekends with her friends or on weekdays after work with her co-workers, she knows she has to change that part of her life immediately to prepare to deliver a healthy baby. If she wasn't taking vitamins prior to her pregnancy she knows she has to create a new daily routine to take prenatal vitamins and any other supplements suggested by her doctor to support the development of her unborn child. When something is growing inside of you it's necessary to breathe life into it. A woman knows not to get in a physical altercation during her pregnancy because there's a great chance that she could lose the baby or cause permanent damage to the development of her child. Although that feeling that lives inside us all keeps growing, personal boundaries should be set to prevent any damage to the outcome of future expectations. Physical altercations, verbal abuse, and threats are examples of the damage we could cause to our purpose that could prevent us from gaining the respect we desperately desire to captivate our communities.

The Day of Birth

The unfortunate part about making a difference is that we aren't always there to witness the change. There are people in this world who spend more time at the doctor's office than they do in their own home. They would rather see themselves deteriorate before investing any time and energy in a clean diet to make a difference in their recovery. There are people involved in the animal agriculture who see the damage their line of work causes to our environment but refuse to make a change to improve the condition of the world we live in. There are circus directors and zoo keepers who take joy in taking animals out of their natural habitat to perform silly acts for the amusement of our children. Our children are being conditioned to believe non-human lives exist for human satisfaction. Giving birth is about applying pressure and pushing. It takes one person to influence many people and many people to influence others.

The stage we're in on this journey doesn't mean the birthing of our future hasn't begun. We are in a time of awareness where things that weren't taught in school are now being taught through social media outlets and other influential platforms. Although we are not equal to non-human lives, we should respect their right to live and thrive in their natural habitat without our interference in their livelihood. Our future is in our hands and how we channel our deepest most passionate aspirations is through unity, love, peace, and understanding.

In Conclusion (Part 3) . . .

Part 3 is about unity and growth. The fight is in full effect and how we continue this journey will reveal the impact we have on future generations. We know firsthand how devastating tragedies are. Facing the reality of a damaged land and a new deadly disease epidemic is unnerving and traumatic. Finding a healthy balance for all living things could save us from a few heartbreaks.

This beautiful world we live in should be valued. It provides our every need for survival. Every plant, herb, and seed is filled with nutrients to keep us alive and well. Our animals shouldn't be used to get what earth has already given us. Using our resources wisely will save our animals and land from enduring the pain and suffering inflicted by our self-serving ways. We have the power to create a new normal for the people of the future. The Amazon, our largest rainforest, has suffered from deforestation. This doesn't just affect our land but all living things. This sets the trajectory of what tragedies future generations might have to endure because of our bad decisions.

Birthing our future is about changing our behavior and living an eco-friendly lifestyle. We have to come to a peaceful common ground by becoming cautious eaters to create better living conditions for all. This fight comes full circle and the animal rights movement is just one part of the fight. Every decision we make creates a domino effect that affects the livelihood of every living thing. Let's make this fight one to remember.

Postscript

Thank you for following your heart and being a great addition to The Vegan Fight. The fact that you've made it to the end of this book shows your eagerness to make a change. Throughout our lives we're continuously learning something new – taking steps to improve the ones we made prior. Remember that you are whatever your heart desires. Always be true to yourself and vow to never betray that trust.

Made in United States
Orlando, FL
07 February 2023

29657074R00096